What Others A

OFF B.

MW01014124

Joel Schnoor is a delightful storyteller. He's also a theologian (even if he says he isn't). *Theology* literally means "God study" and there is practical theology here: devotional journal entries, conversations with God, short-stories engaging the everyday miracles of life and the questions left unanswered.

As I read *Off Balance*, I learned, laughed, smiled, cried and reflected. Then I found myself giving thanks to God for life, love, friendship, family, the church and the peace that passes all understanding. This book is an honest gift from a grace-filled and joyful fellow traveler on the road of life.

> *Rev. Kelly Lyn Logue, Pastor*
> *Holly Springs United Methodist Church,*
> *Holly Springs, North Carolina*

Joel's writing is warm, witty, and most of all, wise. Walk with him through the pages of this book and find yourself blessed! Here is living water for the arid places in your life. You will find hope here!

> *Rev. Ray Broadwell, Sr. Pastor*
> *White Plains United Methodist Church,*
> *Cary, North Carolina*

What do you do when life sends an inexplicable circumstance your way—unexpected doesn't begin to describe it—such as a life-altering, potentially life-shattering diagnosis at 38 years of age with four children and you're the primary breadwinner? You try to connect the dots, because if you can find a context, some purpose, some non-apparent good that can come from what life has sent you, you can find it, if not less painful, at least endurable.

Bad things happen to good people, not because we're necessarily bad ourselves, but because our world is fallen. In Joel's case, even when his life seems to be off balance, he stumbles forward to find hope through prayer in the presence of God and in His work, knowing that utimately God will complete our redemption and all that is wrong will cease to be.

Joel's is a moving faith journey that goes beyond his own story to give a divine context for all of us who suffer the inexplicable. It gives us hope while we stumble forward to all things new. Thank you, Joel, for helping us connect the dots.

Rev. Ken L. Milliken, Sr. Pastor
Gospel Tabernacle Church, Dunn, North Carolina

Off Balance

Getting Back Up When Life Knocks You Down

Joel Schnoor

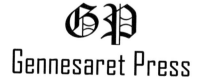

Gennesaret Press

Gennesaret Press
202 Persimmon Place
Apex, NC 27523

www.GennesaretPress.com

ISBN: 978-0-9845541-2-6

Library of Congress Control Number: 2011926260

Printed in the United States of America
Apex, North Carolina

Cover design and illustration by Ken High

To my grandmothers

Susan Blanche (Stevens) Berry

and

Ferne Antoinette (Stember) Schnoor

Table of Contents

Acknowledgements

It is impossible to adequately thank all the people who played a role in the shaping of *Off Balance*. The words that you will read here are from my heart, and my proofreaders and sounding boards have been instrumental in holding me accountable so that what you read is what I really intended.

To all of you who spent time encouraging me, or listening to my ideas, or proofreading and editing this book, thank you!

My parents, Jay and Connie Schnoor, provided me with a safe haven and a happy childhood with two loving siblings, Jennie and Barry. Mom and Dad created a foundation based on joy and love that stayed with me long after I left home, and I believe that provided stability that came in useful later in life.

My two grandmothers, Susan Blanche Berry and Ferne Antoinette Schnoor, played monumental roles in inspiring me. They showed me what it means to get back up on my feet after getting knocked down, and their influence is felt, page after page, throughout the book.

Finally, my Lord and Savior, Jesus Christ, deserves any praise associated with this book. If you are encouraged, inspired, or drawn closer to him, it is his doing, not mine. Both my enthusiasm for life and my tendency to see the humor in everything are traits that are God-given. If this book brings a warm smile to your face, thank him, not me. It is my prayer that you are blessed by what you are about to read.

Joel Schnoor

Psalm 63

Oh God, you are my God,
earnestly I seek you;
my soul thirsts for you,
my body longs for you,
in a dry and weary land
where there is no water.

I have seen you in the sanctuary and
beheld your power and your glory.
Because your love is better than life,
my lips will glorify you.

I will praise you as long as I live, and
in your name I will lift up my hands.
My soul will be satisfied as with the richest of foods;
with singing lips my mouth will praise you.

On my bed I remember you; I think of you
through the watches of the night.

Because you are my help, I sing
in the shadow of your wings.
My soul clings to you; your right hand upholds me.

They who seek my life will be destroyed;
they will go down to the depths of the earth.

They will be given over to the sword and
become food for jackals.

But the king will rejoice in God;
all who swear by God's name will praise him,
while the mouths of liars will be silenced.
                                    —Psalm 63 NIV

Preface

Those who wish to sing always find a song.
Anonymous

The clock has just struck 12:30am, and the mood to write is settling in like an old, affection-starved cat. The rest of the household is fast asleep, but when that creative feeling comes—when I start wading in the ebb and flow of words on the beaches of my mind—I have little choice but to obey its whims and demands. "Don't even think about going to bed now," I tell myself. "Just write like crazy."

This is the story of my faith journey as I try to deal with a chronic illness. This is not a disease-centric book, however. The hope is that this will be helpful to anyone who is hurting for any reason.

The book focuses on several themes that I believe are important aspects of faith and life. I have included humorous stories from my childhood, youth, and young adulthood that tie in with these themes. I have also included entries from my journal, logging the days shortly before and after my brain surgery in 2010 as part of a clinical trial for my illness.

Why did I include humorous childhood stories? Our attitudes, our approaches to life, and our value systems are influenced by experiences from our youth. God doesn't shape a person all at once, and God certainly doesn't wait until we are 18 years old before he starts touching our lives. The experiences of our childhood, youth, and young adulthood—and perhaps events that happened in our parents' and grandparents' lives as well—all play together in determining who we become.

Besides, if you're like me, maybe you want a chuckle, something to ease the pain. Maybe you want to get ideas on how to deal with whatever is tormenting you; your nemesis, named or unnamed, slithers along the floor, hiding under the couch or your bed, waiting for just the right moment to rear its ugly head.

Are there monsters in your closet? Not likely. But it IS likely that you've got your mind on something. What is it?

Maybe it's breast cancer, and you're scared. After all, you're only 42 and you have things to do; you've got plans; you've got mouths to feed and a retirement savings to protect. Or maybe you just learned that you have prostate cancer, and the news rocked your world because your daughter is carrying your first grandchild, and you have been so looking forward to bouncing that baby on your knee and teaching him everything you know about football.

It could be AIDS, lymphoma, Alzheimer's, Multiple Sclerosis, Parkinson's Disease, Clinical Depression, or a host of other things. Maybe the thing troubling you is an addiction that you can't shake— alcohol, tobacco, or other drugs. Maybe you have a personality disorder of some kind. Or maybe you're just having a bad day.

I'm not a theologian; I'm not a doctor; and I'm not a magician who can come in with smoke and mirrors to dazzle you.

I'm like you. A nemesis that I can't seem to shake is stalking me. Will God heal and restore me in my lifetime? Maybe. For whatever reason, God has not chosen to lift this burden from me—yet. However, I can tell you right now that God is enabling me to live with joy and a sense of peace that can't come from anywhere but him.

There are a lot of *maybes* on this page. Will this book be helpful? Maybe. That's my goal. If nothing else happens, I hope you at least take a look at Psalm 63 tonight. In fact, try reading Psalm 63 several times a day for a week.

Will my writing encourage you? Will you feel a bit uplifted?

Maybe. That's my prayer, anyway—that anyone who reads this book will find something to make him or her smile, something to bring him or her a little closer to God, and something that can be shared with a friend or anyone else in need.

Anyway, we're burning daylight. Let's get started!

Joel Schnoor
March 2011

Timing the Punch Line

Standing in the aisle near the back row, with the audience seated around him, the comedian turned to a rather innocuous-looking man wearing gray slacks and a dark blue sport coat. The seated man looked apprehensive, not sure what to expect.

"I want you to ask me two questions," said the comedian. "First, I want you to ask me what I do for a living. Then, I want you to ask me what is my greatest challenge with my job."

The man in the dark blue coat smiled. Apparently he felt that this seemed simple enough. "Okay," he began, "what do you do for a living?"

"I'm a stand up comedian," said the stand up comedian.

"And what is your greatest—" continued the man.

"Timing," said the comedian, interrupting the man.

"—challenge with your job," said the man, finishing his sentence and looking befuddled.

In any story, timing is everything.

My story is part of a larger picture that spans generations, but the outcome is already different in my time than it was for one of my grandparents.

Advances in the understanding of human anatomy and medicine have led to curing disease and eradicating illness. For example, not that long ago a diagnosis of smallpox meant death or disfigurement; today, smallpox is almost nonexistent. Does this mean that life was unfair for the thousands who died of smallpox in the past?

It would be too easy to write that we should accept the things that happen to us within our generational boundaries and just move on. Your great-grandfather may have died from an illness that you cannot contract, and you may die from an illness that your great-grandchildren will not be able to contract.

The topic of illness touches everybody, and volumes have been written that try to rationalize why bad things happen to good people. Theologically and philosophically, what does it all mean? Is life fair? Is it supposed to be?

Within the spans of our lives, we start out as fearless little kids, and then we gradually progress into adulthood, where we end up as cynics crying out that life is cruel and unfair. A job loss, a broken relationship, an unexpected death in the family—these can all weigh us down and turn our outlook on life into a sad drudgery of unfortunate events.

At some point, though, we discover that we have choices to make. The context of how we live our lives—the foundation for our priorities, our attitudes, and our enjoyment of life—is critical in determining how we handle illness, hardship, pain, and suffering. Where do you put your faith? Where do you put your trust? Are you trying to blaze your own trail toward a joyful life, or has that path already been paved?

Anyway, in the telling of any story, timing is everything. Whodunnits don't typically start out by telling the reader who the murderer is; sporting events don't start out by revealing who the winner will be. In my story, it's not the ending that is interesting—it's the journey itself. The ending needs to be stated up front so that the rest of the story can be cast in that hue.

See, it goes like this. I embrace life. Each morning I look forward to getting out of bed and starting the day. It reminds me a little of comedian Red Skelton, who summed it up nicely when he said that upon awakening, if a sheet wasn't covering his head and candles weren't burning in the room, he knew it was going to be a great day.

It's easy for someone who embraces life to say that you should embrace life. How does one who doesn't wake up happy each morning, one who tends to have a gloomier outlook, shift gears?

Two key ingredients—a trust in God and a sense of humor—carry a person through the tough times. I contend, actually, that in times of trial it is nearly impossible to see the humorous side of life without having a trust in God.

Life experiences—those anecdotes that happened to you as a child, youth, or adult—can make for funny stories, but they can also help set the stage further down the road. Cherish those moments. Bask in the knowledge that the adventure making you cringe right now may be funny in five years or, at least, that it may be helpful in dealing with some crisis that comes along.

Consider this: I have one kid in college and three in high school or middle school; I have a loving, supportive wife and a wonderful extended family; I have undergraduate and graduate degrees in one of the hottest fields (Computer Science) in the world; and I already have one book published and several others in progress. You probably wouldn't be surprised if you found me praising God, enjoying life, and writing that we shouldn't spend our time worrying. You might be inclined to think that I have it all together.

You would be wrong. Now it's time for the punch line.

I was diagnosed on September 13, 1999 with Parkinson's Disease. I was thirty-eight years old.

I

Worry and a Psalm 63 Context

Do not be afraid of tomorrow, for God is already there.

Anonymous

Do not worry about whether or not the sun will rise.
Be prepared to enjoy it.

Anonymous

February 20, 2010

*T*en days from now, it will either happen or it won't. I guess you already knew that. On March 2nd, 2010, I will either have brain surgery or I won't.

If it happens—if the needles shall pierce this God-made brain of mine—then I will see one of three things. First, the hope is that there will be some relief from this insidious illness, either large or small. I'm praying for a miracle and that Parkinson's will be fast removed from my being.

Second, it's possible there will be complications or that side effects will be worse than any benefit from the gene therapy. Changes in personality, shifts in obsessive behavior, and things like that could result.

Finally, there could be no change at all. I almost see that as the most unlikely scenario, given what will be contained in the injection.

Injection? Wait, back up.

For Parkinson's Disease (PD), the whole deal is about dopamine, the chemical in the brain that triggers the body's movement. Every move a body makes—walking, swinging the arms, tying a knot, throwing a ball, chewing, swallowing, talking, etc.—depends on dopamine. When PD symptoms begin appearing, the person with PD has already lost 80% of those dopamine-producing neurons.

In the CERE-120-09 clinical trial for Parkinson's Disease, the basic idea is that a virus containing the protein neurturin will be injected into my brain (specifically, into two regions of the brain known as the putamen and the substantia nigra, where most dopamine-producing neurons live) through two holes, approximately one inch diameter each. In the laboratory, neurturin has been shown to repair and restore the damaged dopamine-producing neurons in rats.

I am to be the third of six people in Phase One (the "safety and efficacy" phase) who will receive the surgery and then be closely monitored to make sure it's reasonably safe, before the trial is opened to a larger group of participants.

That almost boggles my mind.

If this works, it will be the first time that anything has been found to reverse, stop, or even slow down the progression of this disease. We can pray for that. Am I excited? Sure. Worried? No. Is God in charge of this? You bet.

The First Sled Ride

When I was two, our family moved to La Crescent, Minnesota, a hilly, picturesque town nestled along the Mississippi River in apple orchard country. We rented a house at the top of one of the town's several hills, and in front of the house the street rolled downward and downward and downward before leveling off into a nice straight run where it then crossed Elm Street and a couple of other streets before heading on out of town.

On a snowy day that winter, Dad thought it was high time to take me out for my first sled ride.

He bundled me up in layers of pants, shirts, sweaters, and socks. After all, at my tender age, he wanted to make sure I'd be safe from catching a cold. He put snow boots on my feet, buried me in a sky blue fuzzy coat, put a stocking cap on my head, and put warm wool mittens on my hands. I was ready!

We walked to the crest of the hill. Dad set the sled down, oriented it in the right direction, and placed me on it. All he had to do was finish getting ready himself. As he pulled on his gloves, he probably glanced up at the apple orchards in the hills above the house, admiring the beauty of the fresh snowfall.

As he finished his preparation, his thoughts were interrupted with the excited yell of a little voice that was quickly growing more distant. Dad looked down at his feet. The sled was gone! He looked down the street. The sled was zooming downhill, straight as an arrow, and I was sitting on top, a little bundle of blue flying at breakneck speed.

Dad might have set a human land speed record as he sprinted down the hill, trying to catch the sled. As he ran, he was probably praying for three things: first, that the sled would continue a straight path, avoiding the cars parked along the side; second, that the sled wouldn't get hit by any cars as it crossed Elm Street; and third, that Mom wouldn't kill him when she found out what had happened.

The first two prayers were answered on the spot. The sled ran a perfectly straight course down the center of the street, leveling off at the bottom of the hill and then flying through the Elm Street intersection unscathed, finally stopping just before the next intersection.

Anyway, when Dad reached me, he found me laughing and saying, "Again, Daddy, again. Again please."

The third prayer was also answered (at least as of this writing).

It's interesting that it was the adult in this story who was scared. I was too naive to know I should be afraid—or was I? Perhaps my simple, childlike trust was the way it was supposed to be, at least back in Genesis before Adam and Eve disobeyed God and fell into sin.

Why do we worry about anything? Man was not designed to worry. Adam feared nothing until he had sinned (Genesis 3:10). God wants us to trust him, to lean on him completely. What's preventing us from doing that?

The Surprise Party

When my brother Barry was about to turn two years old, my sister Jennie and I (aged four and almost six, respectively) decided that we would have a surprise party for him. Jennie and I walked around the neighborhood, inviting friends and getting everything planned. The party was to be Saturday at 3pm.

Our invitation list had twenty names of people who had said they would come.

Jennie and I were excited for the big day—it was the first time we had planned anything like this—and we worked hard to keep it a secret.

We came up with a list of games to play and even had a plan in case it rained. We got all of our outside toys ready in case the weather was good, and we got all of our inside toys ready in case the weather was bad.

On the day of the party, we were doing the final cleanup of the living room, and Mom walked in.

"Why, you're doing a great job cleaning!"

"Thanks, Mom. Just getting ready for the party," said my sister.

"Party?" said Mom.

At that moment, Jennie and I looked at each other with an I-thought-you-told-her kind of a look.

"Uh, um, yes, we're having a surprise party for Barry."

Mom looked a little on edge. She asked, "What time is the party?"

"Three o'clock today."

"Fifteen minutes from now?"

"Oh," I said, looking at the clock, "yeah, I guess so."

"How many people are you expecting?"

"Oh, um, twenty people said they could come."

In the blink of an eye, Mom shoved a few dollars into my fist and commanded, "Run to the store and get two cartons of ice cream!" She raced into the kitchen and began baking a batch of brownies.

Jen and I high-tailed it down the street to the corner store. The store clerk greeted us as we ran in, and he said, "Your mom just called. She wants you to get some candles too." Fortunately, we had enough money.

We grabbed the ice cream and candles and ran back up the hill toward home. By the time we got home, the first guests had already arrived. Mom could have been flustered by the surprise, but instead we saw a smile on her face.

Life catches us off-guard, and even happy events can surprise us. If we get upset at the little things, there is no way we will be able to handle the big things. Mom showed me that it is possible to respond with grace when our own plans and priorities get interrupted or supplanted unexpectedly.

Day One

On my first day of first grade, I dutifully found my name on the class roster in the hallway and I reported to the appropriate classroom. My kindergarten teacher the year before had been young and pretty with a big smile. I expected more of the same.

Mrs. Wilson walked into the room. She was not young; she was not pretty; and she was not smiling. She began by saying that we first would have introductions and we would come to the front of the class one at a time as she announced our names. She eventually called, "Joel." I immediately stood up and walked to the front of the class. To my surprise, another boy also stood up and walked to the front of the class. He looked equally perplexed.

Mrs. Wilson scowled and then hissed, "Which of you is Joel Moore?" The other boy raised his hand.

Looking me in the eye, Mrs. Wilson snarled, "What are you doing up here? Sit down!" She grabbed me by the shoulders, turned me around, and delivered a swift boot on my bottom, sending me flying across the room. I sat down, humiliated and longing for kindergarten.

A few kids later, she deliberately and slowly said, "Joel," looking at me. I sat for a few seconds to see if yet another Joel might be lurking in the room. No one else stood. "Joel, come here," she roared, looking straight at me. I meekly obeyed, feeling like a whipped puppy who didn't quite understand what he had done wrong.

The next three hours passed without further incident. At lunch time, though, Mrs. Wilson issued the orders: those who brought lunch, line up on the left; those with meal tickets, line up on the right. Each child stood and got in line. Each child except me, that is. I was the only one still sitting. I hadn't brought a lunch, and I knew nothing about a meal ticket. Mrs. Wilson marched all the kids out of the room, and I was wondering what to do next.

I sat there for a minute or two, my heart racing. Should I go follow Mrs. Wilson? I stood up and poked my head out into the hallway. Nobody was there. I didn't know where the cafeteria was, either. I did what any six-year-old kid would do in that situation. I panicked. I raced home, bursting through the front door.

This startled Mom, who had been in the kitchen doing motherly things. "What's wrong?" she asked. I explained about the lunch dilemma. It turned out that Mom had indeed bought a meal ticket for me.

Mom graciously cooked a box of macaroni and cheese and then told me she was going to drive me back to school. I wasn't thrilled about the prospect of setting foot in that building again. Even though I was reluctant to get in the car, I did. However, when we arrived and Mom got out of the car, I performed the most brilliantly defiant act of my tender age. I locked all the car doors. I was still inside the car.

Mom pleaded with me to come out of the car. No way. I was done with first grade. It wasn't for me. On the playground, Mom found a friend of mine who came over and tried to convince me to get out of the car. I was crying, and a crowd gathered around the car. Finally, I relented. I'm not sure why.

I walked into the school, found my seat in the classroom, and a moment later Mrs. Wilson returned. The first words out of her mouth were, "Did you hear about the cry baby who locked himself in the car and wouldn't come out?" All eyes—Mrs. Wilson's too—turned to me.

That was my first day of first grade, and it was the first time I had ever experienced the kind of disappointment that sent me reeling, doubting myself. I began worrying.

I think I noticed my first gray hair that evening. It was a long year.

Worry (Who's in Charge Here, Anyway?)

Thousands gathered on the hillside to listen to this man, a carpenter's son from Nazareth. They came from miles around to hear him; people said there was something different about him. He spoke a new set of words; his eyes showed compassion for the people, not the fierce war-like menacing look that most of the other would-be messiahs had revealed through the years.

He spoke softly, and his words turned the world on its head. He said that being angry at someone is as bad as murder; looking at someone with a lustful eye is as bad as adultery; and that instead of an eye for an eye, we should not resist an evil enemy. He also said do not worry.

> Then Jesus said to his disciples: "Therefore I tell you,
> do not worry about your life, what you will eat;
> or about your body, what you will wear.
> Life is more than food, and the body more than clothes.
> Consider the ravens: They do not sow or reap, they have
> no storeroom or barn; yet God feeds them.
> And how much more valuable you are than birds!
> Who of you by worrying can add a single hour to his life?
> Since you cannot do this very little thing, why do you
> worry about the rest?"
>
> —Luke 12:22–26

In Matthew he adds:

> Therefore do not worry about tomorrow,
> for tomorrow will worry about itself. Each
> day has enough trouble of its own.
>
> —Matthew 6:34

Do you remember the things that made you anxious as a child? Maybe you worried about whether you would be picked last for the kickball game during school recess; or whether your friend would trade you his Hank Aaron card without you having to give up your Willie Mays card; or whether your favorite team would win its next game; or whether the girl with brown hair who sat in the front row at school liked you as much as you thought you liked her.

Then, more or less suddenly, your voice started changing, you found hair growing in your armpits, and Dad told you that he needed you to work at the lumber yard this Saturday and perhaps every Saturday after that. You agreed to it, but inside you were cringing with remorse because the end of those carefree days had come. The Saturday job quickly turned into an every-day-all-summer-long job. Never again would you play catch or go fishing with your best friend in the early morning sun. Your bare feet, used to running in the grassy meadows, were laced up with heavy work boots. Your carefree bounce had been superseded by the calculated swagger of a young man knowing he was beginning to earn real money.

Perhaps most significant of all, the things you worried about "grew up." Instead of baseball cards, you found yourself thinking about gas money and auto insurance. Instead of playing catch with the boy next door, you had your eye on the girl down the street for the school homecoming dance. You started thinking about universities and getting your grades up, and before you knew it, you were preparing to graduate from college and you were hunting for a job.

Soon you were thinking about how to get food on the table to feed your kids; how to provide adequate health care coverage; and which cell phone plan was the best for your family. You started planning for retirement and began saving a nest egg. You also started worrying more about aches and pains and unidentified lumps that appeared in awkward places on your body.

Even if you excelled in all that planning, you may have started worrying about the meaning of life. After all, you were in your mid-fifties; had you accomplished anything that would last, something of eternal value?

Why do we worry? Oh, I know the answer. "It's only natural to worry."

Is it really? If we didn't worry as children because we knew that our parents (who were not perfect) would provide, does it make sense to worry as adults when we (should) know that God (who is perfect) will provide?

"Well yeah," you argue, "but I'm responsible for my family." So, we worry about making ends meet. We worry whether we have overlooked something in planning for college or for retirement.

Of course you are responsible for your family. God does want us to manage what he gives us wisely. He wants us to be good stewards. He also wants us to trust him.

See, we may not know how every day is going to play out. In the long run, though, we already know the outcome. The Bible tells us the end of the story. We know who's going to win the game. Yet we still worry. I believe God wants us to be diligent but that he also wants us to forget about worrying.

Think of it like this. Your alma mater is about to play for the college football national championship. You are a nervous wreck, perhaps, and will continue to be on edge until the outcome of the game is well in hand. Because your team has so much on the line, you can't really relax and enjoy the game.

In the 1996 Fiesta Bowl, the Nebraska Cornhuskers went up against the Florida Gators for the national championship. Going into the game, Nebraska was ranked #1 in the polls and Florida was #2. Behind quarterback Tommie Frazier, Nebraska had a powerful offense that season; Florida's offense was explosive, however, and could score points in a hurry.

As a Nebraska alum and a long time Nebraska football fan, I was anxious at the beginning of the game. I knew that Florida would be tough, and after the opening quarter of play, Nebraska was behind 10-6. Well, the Husker offense erupted in the second quarter; the Husker defense shut down the Gators; and Nebraska took a 35-10 lead into the locker room at halftime.

Early in the third quarter, Nebraska scored again to take a 42-10 lead. The Nebraska announcers began proclaiming victory, even though time-wise there was still a lot of football to play.

Although the game was far from over time-wise, the rejoicing had begun. Husker fans ceased worrying, knowing who was going to win the game.

It's this way with Jesus. He has already won the battle. He died on the cross for our sins, and then he overcame death with the resurrection. There is no question who is going to win the battle, because it is done. This battle isn't just a football game. This is real life.

"But what about life's daily battles?" you ask. We live in a fallen world, where there is sickness and death and pain and suffering. Is it really possible in modern society to not be anxious about anything? Is that doable in today's world? With concerns about the economy and joblessness and everything else, the Bible still calls us to rejoice always. Always is a long time.

Worry can paralyze you; worry can draw your attention away from God, your source of strength and help, and cause you to want to solve everything yourself. Worrying about something will not make the problem go away; in fact, it could make things worse because it affects your words and your actions.

When was the last time you exhibited the child-like certainty that God really is in control and that he knows what he's doing? This isn't a mind game; this isn't some psychological trick to talk yourself into feeling better. This requires a commitment on a daily basis to turn to God, to ask for his help, and to leave your worries at his feet.

My life is in God's hands. These are the hands that created the heavens and the earth. These are the hands that healed the paralyzed, the hands that put mud in the eyes of a blind man and gave him sight. These are the hands that were pierced on the cross—for me. These hands are capable enough for me!

The surgery is only days away, and it's all in God's hands. Surgery! I always wondered when my first hospital stay would be. This is voluntary—entirely—and yet this is a glimmer of hope for being able to play with my kids for many more years; for being able to play with my grandkids; for being able to travel and enjoy retirement; and for living the active life I desire.

This is the rainbow! What lies at the other end? I don't know, but it is reason for hope.

The love I have received from the folks at White Plains United Methodist Church has been amazing! Of course, this is the way the Body of Christ should be. This should be the norm. This is the type of love and support I would expect from a perfect world.

The world is not perfect, nor is White Plains, but with a focus on Christ I think this church is going to be about as close as we can get to showing God's love, short of heaven.

Lord I love you. Thank you for putting us here at White Plains.

The desire to be afraid, the tendency to bathe in fear, creeps under the doorway like a serpent hunting its prey. To be in charge, to have control, is really what we seek.

How dare God put my well-being in someone else's hands! A person I have only met once is going to open up my brain.

But wait—who is really in charge here? This same God who created the universe, who counts the lilies of the field, is the same God who made us. He knows how to guide the surgeon's hands.

Lord, help me keep you at the center of my life.

The experience certainly will give me time to reflect on the role that Parkinson's Disease has played in my life, both as an adult and as a youth. After all, I am not the first in my family to have to deal with Parkinson's Disease.

Grandma

Rewind several decades to a cold Sunday morning in January of 1974 in Onawa, Iowa, nestled between the Loess Hills and the Missouri River, where we lived with my maternal grandmother.

"I would like to stay home this morning and watch Grandma," I exclaimed.

"Me too!" shouted my little sister and little brother in unison.

Our parents agreed that all three of us could stay home from church to be with Grandma on that cold winter day. It didn't matter that we were only twelve, ten, and eight years old, respectively. If a problem came up, church was only a block and a half away.

"Remember, you're staying home to be with Grandma. No TV unless Grandma wants to watch," Mom reminded us. She and Dad headed out the door.

Barry stayed in the room with Grandma while Jen and I went into the kitchen to make breakfast. Minutes later, we carried a tray with a bowl of oatmeal and a glass of orange juice into Grandma's room. One of us—I don't remember which one—fed Grandma with a spoon. She ate six or seven bites and then she pointed to the orange juice. I lifted the glass and she drank a sip with a straw. Jen wiped Grandma's chin with a napkin, removing a small stream of juice that had dribbled back out of Grandma's mouth.

Grandma asked if we could read the Bible to her. She especially loved the book of John, so we read the first chapter. Then Jennie asked her to tell us a story.

"Once upon a time, when I was a little girl," began Grandma in a whisper, as we kids gathered on the floor around her, "I made a little bag of raisins to take to my teacher at the one-room schoolhouse."

Grandma paused to catch her breath. She spoke with a stutter, and her speech was often reduced to a barely audible whisper.

We kids listened intently and patiently.

Grandma continued. "My friend Maidie came to my house so that we could walk to school together, and we stopped by the little rabbit hutch out back to visit my new pet rabbit on the way."

Again she paused, pointing to the glass of orange juice.

One of us raised the orange juice to Grandma's mouth, and she took another sip through the straw. Again, a little bit of juice ran down her chin, and again we wiped it with a napkin.

"I had another bag with me, and Maidie and I scooped a few of the rabbit droppings—they looked like pellets and were the same color as raisins—and we put them in the bag."

There was a long pause, and we soon realized that Grandma had dozed off. The last couple of years had been like that. Grandma would wear down so quickly, like an old battery that couldn't hold its charge. In those two years that we had lived with her, the change had been dramatic. Everything was slow paced. Grandma had problems eating; she had a hard time talking; she had difficulty walking and keeping her balance; and everything she did seemed to be in slow motion, kind of like watching football replays on television.

Grandma had Parkinson's Disease.

In the 1970s, telling a person that he or she had Parkinson's Disease was a death knell. The medical community did not know how to combat the symptoms effectively, and we now know that the treatments most commonly used at the time did more damage to the body than the disease itself.

Grandma wore a wig because the medicine had made all of her hair fall out. Even though she had long stopped leaving the house for social events, Grandma maintained her dignity and tried to look presentable every day, choosing to get dressed and putting on her makeup.

When she woke up from her nap a few minutes later, she continued. "We got to school, and Sally Slaughter saw us coming. She was as mean as a hornet. She walked up to me and pushed me to the ground. The two bags fell out of my pocket, and Sally picked them up and ran off."

"Oh no!" my sister exclaimed. "That wasn't nice."

Grandma laughed. "No, it wasn't nice. Anyway, class began, and when our teacher Mrs. Baines walked in, Sally stood up and said, 'Mrs. Baines, I brought in some raisins for you.' Sally gave Mrs. Baines one of the bags."

"Which bag did Mrs. Baines get?" asked my brother.

"Well," continued Grandma, "during lunch we were all outside in the sunshine, and Sally opened the remaining bag, poured some of its contents into her hand, and popped them into her mouth."

We eagerly waited in anticipation to hear what happened next.

"I need to stand up," said Grandma.

"Sure, Grandma," we said, all three of us helping her out of her chair. She stood for a minute or so and seemed to have her balance, so we let go. That was a mistake. She fell backward, but fortunately her chair was there. She landed hard on the seat, snapping her head back and sending her wig flying across the room.

"Grandma, are you okay!" I exclaimed.

There was a pause, and then she broke into laughter. It was a soft laughter but it came from her heart.

"Yes, I'm okay," she whispered. She continued laughing, and soon all of us were laughing.

My brother retrieved the wig and we tried to put it on her head, but we weren't really successful with that. It was lopsided and lumpy. We brought a mirror to Grandma, and she laughed even harder.

"Grandma, could you finish the story please?" asked my sister.

"Story?" asked Grandma.

"You know, about the raisins and the rabbit and Susan Slaughter."

"Oh yes, the raisins," said Grandma. "Well, Susan put a handful of them into her mouth, only they weren't really raisins."

"Oh no!" cried my brother, smiling.

"Oh yes," said Grandma, also smiling. It was unusual to see her smile. Parkinson's Disease had changed her face so that her expression was usually frozen—this is called the Parkinson's Mask—and it was hard to tell just by looking at her whether she was happy.

"What happened then?" I asked.

"Susan spat them out and tried wiping her tongue with her shirt sleeve. She turned green and ran behind the school for a few minutes."

"So Mrs. Baines really got raisins," said my sister.

"Yes, but Susan didn't know that," said Grandma, "and she was worried all afternoon that Mrs. Baines would open the bag and begin eating them."

"Grandma," asked my sister, "what were you going to do with the rabbit droppings anyway?"

But Grandma had dozed off again, or perhaps she just pretended to sleep. Either way, we never did find out the answer to that question.

She slept until lunch. I didn't know if it was the disease or all the medication that made her so tired. I knew one thing though. Grandma always had a cheerful disposition, never complaining, never fussing, always exhibiting joy in the face of adversity.

God was at the center of Grandma's life. Not only did Grandma read the Bible and spend time in prayer—and she found great comfort in that—but she had the courage to humble herself before God, to acknowledge that he was in charge, not she. Grandma knew that God's plan for her was the perfect plan. She had hope that after her life on earth had passed, things on the other side would be better.

Candles

One Saturday afternoon in the early spring of 1974, I sat home alone in the house with Grandma. Watching television in the den, I barely noticed her shuffling through the hallway and down the short flight of steps into the living room. Then I heard the piano. I don't remember the piece—I hadn't heard it before—but its beauty struck me. The delicate touch of the keys testified to the expertise of the pianist as well. Who was playing? I knew Mom and Dad weren't home, nor were my siblings. I ran down the steps into the living room, only to find Grandma sitting there, her withered hands gracefully playing on the keyboard.

"Grandma, that's beautiful!" I exclaimed.

"Isn't it?" she agreed in a matter of fact way, not with pride but with the fondness with which one would acknowledge an old, loyal friend.

"I wish you could play more often, Grandma," I suggested.

"So do I, Joel," she whispered. "So do I." She closed the lid to the keyboard. That was the last time she played.

She was at peace with the fact that she could no longer easily do the things she had once mastered.

As Grandma's disease progressed, the doctors ramped up her medication levels until her body just couldn't take any more, and eventually she experienced liver and kidney failure. On September 6, 1974, I came home from a junior high school football game only to find the candles burning and my mother sobbing. Grandma had passed away.

The two year period living with Grandma was the first—and for many years, the only—experience I had with Parkinson's. I witnessed the ruthless nature of this disease, an illness that robbed my grandmother of the last few productive years of her life. That tragedy was not lost on me. I also saw, though, the tenacity of a fighter refusing to go down. This "old person's disease" took its toll on Grandma's body, but it never touched her spirit. She remained joyful and at peace through the end. I didn't know it at the time, but her response to Parkinson's Disease would be a model for me to follow, years later.

Choices and a Psalm 63 Context

What are the most important things in your life? What makes you happy?

It's all about context, isn't it? When the walls in your world are getting knocked down—when the big, bad wolf comes and blows down your house along with everything you've been trying to save for years—where does your hope rest? Are you anchored firmly on the rock, or are you tied up to a piece of driftwood that is floating along with you?

Why does your context really matter? Simply put, something that is important in one context may have no relevance in another.

After my dad finished his rotation in the Navy, he went to grad school in the Midwest. I was two years old at the time, and with my little sister having just been born and my parents occupied with her, I had some free time on my hands. I enjoyed playing a game that involved removing the contents of dresser drawers and hiding the contents elsewhere. On one particular afternoon, Dad had finished his school work early, so when he came home that night he didn't have to open his briefcase. He didn't open it all evening. I had watched him open it many times, though, and I knew how to do it.

The next day, Dad went to class. The instructor asked the students to turn in their assignments. The man to the left of Dad opened his briefcase—click, click—and pulled out his assignment. The man to the right of Dad opened his briefcase—click, click—and pulled out his assignment. Dad opened his briefcase—click, click—and, with a look of horror, found a black negligee. There was no assignment, no homework, in the briefcase. All he found was just one black negligee.

In the right context, Dad wouldn't have minded seeing the black negligee. But this wasn't the right context.

What's the context by which you live your life? Is health the main thing you think about? I often hear people say, "Well, at least I have my health." Maybe your job—climbing that corporate ladder—defines who you are, and you proudly sacrifice family time as you pursue an additional 1% bonus at the end of the year. Or perhaps your appearance—and a weight-losing, muscle-building, youthful-look-enhancing regimen—rules your schedule.

What if your health goes downhill? What if you lose your job? What if you're stricken with an illness that disfigures you?

My maternal grandmother lived in a world where tremors, drooling, stuttering, and walking with a shuffle were commonplace—a world where her graceful appearance was replaced with balance problems, bradykinesia (slow movement), hair loss, a frozen mask-like appearance, and incontinence. Yet, she had a joy and peace about her that was just amazing. God was at the center of her universe.

I have to contrast that with my great aunt, my grandmother's sister-in-law. Out of respect for family, I don't want to use her real name here, so let me just call her Aunt Cholera. Aunt Cholera lived in Sioux City, Iowa, about 35 miles away from where I grew up in Onawa, Iowa. Aunt Cholera had her health; she had the means of living a comfortable life. She lived independently, with no nursing assistance needed, and she could even drive a car until she died in her mid 80s. Aunt Cholera, though, was living in a different context. She was living in a "me first" context. That meant that if things didn't go her way—and I mean exactly her way—then she would have a fit. She was an adult version of the stereotypical two year old. She was a control freak; she was a manipulator; and boy, Aunt Cholera could throw a tantrum. She could make any child (or any adult for that matter) feel terrible. She thrived on it.

My grandma had Parkinson's Disease, and she watched helplessly as this disease decimated her talents, her health, and eventually her life. Yet, through all of this, Grandma loved life and her faith in God was steadfast. Aunt Cholera had everything, yet she was miserable.

The focal point at the center of your life is a choice. You can't choose the circumstances around you; you can't choose the things that may cause you to struggle. But you can choose the context that defines your priorities and your meaning in life.

So, what are you going to choose? With every day, with every decision, with every encounter with another person, you've got a choice as to how you handle it, how you respond. The good news is that it is your decision. You can choose to be miserable (and make everyone around you miserable) or you can choose to accept the love, joy and peace that God is offering you.

Do you remember really falling in love for the first time? I don't mean a crush or infatuation, but the real thing. Do you remember being so giddy that you didn't eat, you didn't sleep, and the only thing you could do was to dream about being with this other person?

Well, I think that God wants us to be so in love with him, so in love with the life he has given us, that we live each day and each moment with a passion that is even deeper than any love we have felt before.

One of my favorite psalms is Psalm 63, and this illustrates the passion and the yearning for God that I believe he wants us to have. This psalm helps me set my perspective daily.

Oh God, you are my God, earnestly I seek you;
my soul thirsts for you, my body longs for you,
in a dry and weary land where there is no water.

I have seen you in the sanctuary and
beheld your power and your glory.
Because your love is better than life,
my lips will glorify you.

I will praise you as long as I live, and
in your name I will lift up my hands.
My soul will be satisfied as with the richest of foods;
with singing lips my mouth will praise you.

On my bed I remember you; I think of you
through the watches of the night.

Because you are my help, I sing
in the shadow of your wings.
My soul clings to you; your right hand upholds me.

—Psalm 63:1–8

Everybody is dealing with something. It could be broken health; it could be a broken relationship; it could be a broken employment situation; broken finances; or broken anything. It's easy to get discouraged; it's easy to lose sight of what's ultimately important. When we're feeling sad and blue, we need to check our priorities; when the floor seems to drop out from beneath our feet, we need to take a look at our context.

Are you seeking God earnestly? Does your soul thirst for him? Does your body long for him? Are you singing in the shadow of his wings because of his protection and help?

So we're back to where we started. It's all about context, isn't it? It's all about what we surround ourselves with, how we spend our time, where our priorities are, and what things are important to us. On a day-to-day basis, what do we cling to, what do we listen to, what do we watch, what do we think about? Are we satisfied, or are we continually chasing the next thing? Do we live a life dependent on God or are we trying to do it on our own?

You do know who needs to be at the center of your daily life. I encourage you to spend time with him. Live in a Psalm 63 context. Live in a Scriptural context. Live in a God context.

II

Hope and Love

At present we are on the outside ...
the wrong side of the door.
We discern the freshness and purity of morning,
We cannot mingle with the pleasures we see.
But all the pages of the New Testament are rustling
with the rumor that it will not always be so.
Someday, God willing, we shall get "in" ...

C.S. Lewis

March 2, 2010 (Part I: Brain Surgery, Anyone?)

The sky was still dark on March 2, 2010 as my wife and I walked from the parking garage in north Durham toward Duke Hospital. Reaching the first corner before crossing the street, I heard an automated voice coming from the stoplight. The voice said, "Wait," in a low, serious tone.

I turned toward the stoplight and, in the same low, serious tone, I answered, "One hundred ninety pounds."

I chuckled at my joke as the light changed and we crossed the street. My wife said nothing, nor did the other man who was also waiting to cross at the corner. I thought it was funny, anyway.

In spite of my upcoming surgery scheduled for later that morning, I felt light-hearted, mentally nimble, and excited to go ahead and get on with it. I felt good. Though I was approaching the surgery with a sense of humor, the importance of what I was about to undertake was not lost on me.

This was a glimmer of hope, both for me and for the whole Parkinson's community. How will it turn out? I don't know. If it works, we'll rejoice. If it doesn't work (and once the scientists figure out why), we'll still know more about the disease and we'll be one step closer to a cure.

Hope is the catalyst that propels us forward.

After entering Duke Hospital, we walked up to the second floor and found surgical admissions. Checking in, I was given a device that would somehow notify me when it was time for me to report back to the front desk. We sat down. My wife made herself comfortable in the chair and began reading a magazine she had brought. I settled into my chair and opened my notebook to begin writing.

No more than five minutes had passed before the device went off, buzzing, flashing, whirring, and whatever else it was doing.

I walked up to the desk and handed the device to the receptionist. "This thing is broken; either that, or I think my turkey is done," I exclaimed with a smile.

She smiled back, handed me an envelope with papers in it, and directed me to the door for "pre-op," where I was to report for surgery. It was time.

Hope

What is hope? The Webster's New World dictionary's definition of hope includes this:

1. To wish for something with expectation of its fulfillment.
2. To have confidence or trust in something.

It seems to me that there are different levels of hope. There is hope that the lemon meringue pie will turn out. There is hope that we will win the game this weekend. To some extent, though we cannot guarantee the outcome of those events, we can do things to help sway the outcome one direction or the other. If we plan and prepare and read the recipe carefully, we can probably end up with a good lemon meringue pie. If we study our opponent and prepare in practice, we have a better chance of winning the game this weekend.

That's the key word though: chance. To a great extent, the things of this world that we hope for are mere wishes; they aren't things or results that we are certain of attaining. The hope that the world gives us is uncertain. We might hope for wealth or we might hope for good health. Those hopes can vanish into thin air.

In Romans, Paul writes:

And we rejoice in the hope of the glory of God.
Not only so, but we also rejoice in our sufferings,
because we know that suffering produces perseverance;
perseverance, character; and character, hope.
And hope does not disappoint us, because God has
poured out his love into our hearts by
the Holy Spirit, whom he has given us.

—Romans 5:2b–5

We rejoice because our hope as Christians is in God's glory, and we know that this hope is secure. When Jesus died on the cross and was resurrected, the hope became a certainty. Our hope for a future of eternity with God has been sealed. The battle is won.

Another way of saying it is this: God loved us so much that he sent his son to die for us (John 3:16); those who accept Jesus as King of kings and Lord of lords receive the Holy Spirit in their hearts (Romans 8:11) and are saved and given eternal life (Romans 10:9). It's a done deal.

Paul also points out that suffering results in perseverance, which builds character; character results in hope. This hope—which is from God—"does not disappoint us," writes Paul. That's the difference between placing our hope in God rather than placing our hope in things of this world.

For example, the difference between my hope for a cure and my hope for God's glory is that my hope for a cure is not a certainty, but my hope for God's glory is guaranteed—it is certain— and therefore will not disappoint me. If our ultimate hope is focused on anything other than God, we likely will end up disappointed.

How are hope and faith related?

> Now faith is being sure of what we hope for and
> certain of what we do not see.
>
> —Hebrews 11:1

A slight rephrasing says it this way: When we are *certain* that our hope will be met—when we are *sure* that our hope will be met—then we have faith.

Knowing that God's promises are true—having faith in the words Jesus spoke when he said (in John 14) that he is preparing a room for me and (in Matthew 11) that he will give me peace, rest for my soul—propels me. How can I not live with joy, knowing what awaits me?

I have hope that I will live with God eternally; I have hope in my salvation. I am sure that God's promises are true. I am certain that through God's grace I have eternal life with God.

> We continually remember before our God
> and Father your work produced by faith,
> your labor prompted by love,
> and your endurance inspired by hope
> in our Lord Jesus Christ.
>
> —1 Thessalonians 1:3

At the end of 1 Thessalonians 1:3, Paul writes that the hope that is placed in Christ inspires endurance. Endurance means you have the strength to keep going. Hope is what keeps you in the game.

Where do you place your hope? Is it in the things of the world, or is it in Christ? Hope that is placed in the world will disappoint you; it is but a fleeting wish, a dream.

I know that God's promises are true, and my hope rests in that. Hope that is placed in Christ has a rock-solid foundation. It is certain. I can bank on it. The assuredness of that hope inspires me, and it gives me the endurance to keep going.

March 2, 2010 (Part II)

A nurse met me at pre-op, and she took some of my blood and measured my weight and inserted part of the IV mechanism in the back of my hand. Once hooked up, that would allow me to receive the anesthesia and everything else.

It's too bad that I couldn't be fed through those tubes. It's easy to imagine a conversation like the following:

"And what would monsieur like today?"

"Uh, could I have an anesthesia, some antibiotics, and maybe a blueberry smoothie?"

"We have a special on anesthesia and antibiotics. Our anesthesia du jour is very good. We are out of blueberry smoothies though."

The pre-op nurse gave me a choice of Curtain #1, Curtain #2, or Curtain #3. I picked Curtain #2. She told me to step behind Curtain #2, to undress completely, and to put on the attractive and well-tailored hospital gown. I guess that was the grand prize for this round of Let's Make a Brain Surgery.

I donned the gown. Drafty and thin, the gown had two ties in the back that were supposed to fasten together. Finger dexterity is not my strong suit (besides, wasn't this one of the reasons I was having the brain surgery in the first place?), and after several attempts at tying the strings I finally had to give up. The nurse (still on the other side of the curtain) told me to go ahead and climb into the bed and to pull the sheet over me. I knew from hospital television shows that I should pull the sheet all the way over my head, so I did. (Just kidding.)

I told the nurse she could come in. She performed some other preliminary tasks and hooked up the IV.

My wife came back to the pre-op area at that time, and she sat next to the bed and we talked a little; then the physician assistant (PA) joined us. She gave me shots to numb four areas on my head—two on the forehead and two in back—to prepare for mounting a frame that would be used for guiding the needles during surgery.

In a minute or two after the numbing shots to the forehead, my wife exclaimed, "You've got horns!" She grabbed a camera and for the next few minutes I felt as though I were posing for Brain Surgery Illustrated. I didn't see the photos until later, but they revealed two peaks coming out of my forehead—not really tall peaks, but big bumps as though I were a deer about to sprout his first set of antlers—and two more peaks in the back of my head. It was into those four peaks that the frame would be screwed.

Getting the frame in exactly the right position required careful mounting. It had to fit over my nose—no small feat—and it had to be centered just right. The PA worked with a lab technician to set the frame exactly and it reminded me of how we set up our Christmas tree each winter. Our tree stand has four screws to support the tree, and each screw has to be adjusted in or out until the tree is upright and balanced. Similarly, four screws attached the frame to my skull, and each one had to be adjusted until the frame reached the desired position.

The PA then attached a device called a halo to the frame. The halo provides the guides that precisely direct the needles into the brain during surgery. After the PA wheeled me down to the basement, the MRI team made maps showing the precise location of the halo guides in relation to the brain.

The MRI people were great. They treated me like a VIP; they put me at ease; and they made me feel special. Of course, that's part of their job. But they had no idea, really, who I was. In that hospital gown, I could have been a billionaire or I could have been homeless. They treated me the same as they treat all their other patients. Their service is not conditional on anything.

That's the way God's love works. He loves you regardless of who you are, regardless of how you treat him, and regardless of your social status, income, skin color, or anything else. After all, he is your creator. Of course, he wants you to love him, but he will love you either way because his love for you is unconditional.

Only a Hat

Growing up, I was a big Atlanta Braves fan, and I wore my Braves baseball cap everywhere I went, except to school and church. I even wore it to bed at night.

In the summer of 1972, we loaded up our white '68 Olds Cutlass station wagon for a trip from our home in Tennessee to western Iowa to visit my maternal grandmother. We set off early in the morning and drove straight through until dinner time, when we got off the interstate to eat in Peoria, Illinois.

My parents wanted to find an Italian restaurant, and we settled on a place called Angelo's. I was wearing my Braves cap as we walked into the restaurant, and I placed the cap on a hat rack. I knew that I shouldn't wear a cap in a restaurant during dinner.

We ate quickly and climbed back into the car at 6:30pm. We still had another five hours to go, and the station wagon zoomed down the entrance ramp and back onto the interstate, heading west into the setting sun. We all eagerly anticipated seeing Grandma again.

The evening started off as perfect as the day had been—deep blue skies and the radiant yellow-orange sunset set the tone for what we thought would be a smooth, happy journey the rest of the way to Grandma's house. We kids were all getting along, and we sang and laughed as we drove down the highway. When we were about forty-five minutes out of Peoria, I stretched my arms back and ran my fingers through my hair, scratching my scalp for a moment.

Something didn't feel right. My hat—my hat was missing!

"Oh no!" I exclaimed. "I left my cap at Angelo's!"

"Are you sure?" asked Mom. We thoroughly searched the car but found no cap.

As soon as we all agreed that I had left it at Angelo's, I heard the turn signal go click-click-click. Dad pulled off onto the exit ramp, crossed the interstate, and in moments we were heading east, back toward Peoria!

You can guess the rest of the story. We returned to Angelo's, where I found the cap sitting on the hat rack inside the entrance. My blunder added an additional hour and a half to our trip that evening.

Dad never said anything. He could have been mad; he could have reminded me of it for the rest of his life. But he did none of those things. Dad just did what Dad always did. He showed unconditional love for one of his kids. He showed grace when he could have shown frustration or anger. That's just the way he was.

In fact, he's still that way. When I mentioned this story to him a few months ago, he had forgotten about it. See, when Dad went back to Angelo's to get that hat, he didn't do it just so that I would forever love him. He went back and got that hat because he forever loves me.

I should also point out that Mom showed unconditional love here as well. Not once did she argue when Dad turned around, even though it was her mom whom we were going to go visit.

But it seems that society expects the moms of the world to be ever loving, and we don't always hold dads accountable. We should.

Anyway, Dad gave me a glimpse that night of how awesome God's love must really be. Would the average dad go back and get that hat? Maybe not. Would God? Certainly. Would my dad? You betcha.

Chevy Impalas and Cherry Pies

With herculean strength, I opened the school door and stepped outside, carrying a stack of textbooks, notebooks, my marching band uniform, and a 4-valve piston King tuba. With a huff, a puff, and a loud grunt, I had achieved the first step home. By my calculations, I had only 2639 steps remaining.

Zoom! A car passed me. Zoom zoom. Two more cars passed me.

I heard another car approaching. This car didn't zoom though. It slowed down and I heard it pull over to the side of the road.

"Need a ride?" asked a familiar voice.

"Sure Mom, that would be great," I replied.

With some effort, I opened the back of the 1975 metallic green Chevy Impala station wagon, one of the last of the big wagons (it officially seated eight but it had room for about forty). I put everything in the back, and then I walked around to the passenger side and hopped into the front seat.

"Thanks for the ride, Mom. That stuff was getting heavy."

"You had quite a load there."

"Yeah, I was going to tell you that they got the tuba fixed and that I'd be bringing it home, but I forgot."

"How'd your test go?" Mom inquired.

"Oh it went fine. I got mixed up on the lie-lay-laid thing again."

"Hens lay, people lie," Mom reminded me.

"So when I pray, 'Now I lay me down to sleep,' I am really talking about chickens?"

"Well no, it's really a little more complex than that."

"That's what I was afraid of."

At that point we were about a block from home.

"So where have you been?" I asked Mom.

"Oh, I went to the church bake sale."

"Oh cool. Did you find anything good there?"

"Well, I bought that cherry pie for dessert tonight."

I turned around and looked in the back seat.

"Where is it?" I asked.

"You ... didn't see it when you got in the car?"

"Should I have?"

I had one of those sinking feelings, kind of like when you're balanced on the back two legs of a chair and there's a moment when suddenly you realize you're going to tip over but there's nothing you can do about it.

As Mom pulled into the driveway, I lifted my bottom up off the seat and ... right there, beneath where I had been sitting, was a flattened cherry pie. Not only was it flattened, but it was the flattest I had ever seen a pie. Of course, the plastic wrap covering the pie didn't prevent the pie filling from leaking. There was cherry pie filling all over the seat.

At first I was mortified, but Mom laughed so hard throughout the rest of the evening that I couldn't help but see the humor in it. We had no dessert that night, contrary to Mom's original plans, but she loved me anyway. When she could have been frustrated and angry, she instead demonstrated her unconditional love for me.

When moments like this come along—whether you are the one who sat on the pie or the one who was planning on eating the pie—you may as well accept it with humility and appreciate it with humor. First, there is nothing you can do to change the fact that it happened. It happened—make the best of it. Second, you are not perfect. If this is the first time you've heard that, I'm sorry to be the one breaking the news to you. Don't worry, though, because no one else is perfect either. These things are going to happen. Get used to it. Third, something like this really is funny. It's okay to be the source of merriment and mirth, even unwittingly. Besides, it could have been a lot worse. I could have skewered myself on a plate of shish kabobs.

A New Life

I asked Jesus into my heart in the spring of 1975, and at that moment I received an insatiable thirst for God's written word, the Bible. I began devouring its contents. Up until that point in my life, the Bible functioned primarily as a large, intimidating history book that described the births of Judaism and Christianity. I approached the Bible with new eyes and a new heart. It was a half-pound cheeseburger and I was a man who hadn't eaten for two weeks.

Plunging into the Bible filled me with an overwhelming sense of the unconditional love that God has for me. My life changed at that point. God put his hands on the dials that control my patience, joy, and enthusiasm, and he cranked everything up to 11. Of course, he left some things for me to work on, and I sometimes find myself struggling in those areas. Lust and pride come to mind, and I'm sure there are others.

Probably the biggest impact on my life, though, was the hope I felt with Christ. Suddenly, life had meaning; life had a purpose. No longer was I living with the end goal being my happiness in this life here on earth; there was a longer term goal, something in the bigger picture that was more important. I finally understood how my grandmother had seemed so calm and joyful, even in the throes of her last days with Parkinson's Disease.

There were two things that I thought about as I began my new life in Christ. First, I wondered how I would respond if I had to deal with a chronic illness, as my grandmother had suffered. Second, I was afraid to witness to others. My life had been blessed, smooth up to that point. How could I convince people that they needed Christ in their lives? Yes, I had become happier, but I had always been happy. Everyone around me knew it, too.

Grandma had been able to use her pain and physical limitations to glorify God. Personally, I wasn't too keen on the idea of demonstrating my faith through pain and physical limitations. There were other ways to glorify God, I reasoned. Not everyone had to be a martyr, and not everyone had to have something wrong in order to be an effective witness for Christ. How would I respond if I ever had to go through something like that? I was hoping I would never have to find out.

As I went through high school and college, witnessing about the joy and peace that comes through Christ, the stock response I would often hear was, "Well of course you're joyful. You've never suffered; everything has always gone your way; your parents are still married; you've never had to deal with illness; etc."

All that was true. My life had been good; I had been blessed in countless ways. What would happen if my world began falling apart? How would I respond if my life began unraveling before my eyes the same way it had for Job, the Biblical paragon of faith who refused to turn away from God even though he lost everything around him?

I often thought back to how Grandma had celebrated life, even in the grip of the ugly, vicious talons of Parkinson's. Did she have to talk herself into having a positive attitude? Did she have to grit her teeth each morning and say, "All right, I'm going to do this," or did she feel herself girded and supported with God's love?

I had the sneaking suspicion that sooner or later I would find out.

Unconditional Love

God's love for us is unconditional, no doubt about it. It's hard to fathom, sometimes, what that really means, though I've long felt that the love a parent has for a child should be as close a model to unconditional love as we'll find on this planet.

Growing up, did you have that "safe place," a place where you knew the meaning of unconditional love? If you are a father or mother, does your view of your role include giving your children your unconditional love, thus helping them see how much God loves them too?

I could depend on my parents to love me always. I could bank on it. That's pretty neat. Each of my parents gave me a clear picture of what God's unconditional love looks like.

Being with either of my parents always recharges my batteries. I feel their love restore me, and I feel their support encourage me. Time spent with them is like a breath of new life for me. Yes, it is life-giving. How unconditional is that? To spend time with someone and to walk away feeling refreshed, uplifted ... wow, how often does that happen?

That leads me to ask myself this question: Do the people on my regular "contact list" walk away feeling refreshed when they spend time with me, or are they drained and wiped out?

Do I emotionally exhaust people, or do I encourage and lift them up? Do people have to be on their guard around me—on their best behavior—or can they let down their hair, be themselves, and relax? Do I accept people as they are instead of what I want them to be? Do my kids feel as rejuvenated after spending a day with me as I do after spending a day with them?

Unconditional love can look like many things, but if it's not life-giving, is it really working?

So the question you're asking may be something along the lines of this: "How does unconditional love tie into chronic illness?"

That's a good question and I'm glad you asked.

If you believe that God loves you unconditionally, and if you believe that he is in charge and knows what he's doing, then you will know that God is not being malicious; you will know that he is not being petty; and you will know that he wants what is best for you.

God created you; God died for you; God loves you; and God has a plan for you.

III

God's Plans

If you want to make God laugh, tell him your plans.

Woody Allen

God's retirement plan is out of this world.

Anonymous

March 2, 2010 (Part III)

As part of the surgery preparation a week ago, the brain surgeon explained to me that he would email the brain images to two other experts around the country, and in a conference call on the day of surgery they together would determine exactly which halo guides to use, which angles to use for positioning the needles, and how deeply to inject the needles.

After the MRI, I remember being wheeled into the operating room (OR). For some reason I had expected the OR to be a small room, but it was huge. The anesthesiologist came in and said, "You'll be feeling a little sleepy," and he was right. I tried lifting my head to tell him I was feeling sleepy.

The next thing I knew, I heard voices talking in the background. Someone said to me, "The surgery is done! How do you feel, Mr. Schnoor?"

"Never better," I mumbled. I remember only a few blurry images for the next several hours, but I do remember saying, "Never better," frequently.

For some reason, there was trouble finding a room for me, but I remember a male nurse coming to the rescue and working hard to find a place for me to go. He was frustrated that the normal modus operandi wasn't working. The problem was that there were 13 people in recovery and only 2 nurses, or something like that, and one of the nurses had to be with the recovering patients the whole time. Anyway, the nurse found a place for me, and at 11:30pm somebody wheeled me to my room. Finally, I would be able to get some rest.

The nurse hooked me up to a monitor that would beep loudly if my pulse got too low (below 50). Well, running had been one of my primary hobbies over the years, and my normal resting pulse rate still tends to hover around 50 or slightly up from there.

For the next few hours, I would nod off to sleep; my pulse would dip below 50; the machine would go into a beeping frenzy, waking me; a *nurse would rush in to make sure I was okay; and the cycle would start all over again. I didn't get a lot of rest.*

Shouldn't we learn early in our lives that our plans often change mid-stream?

Life has a way of keeping us on our toes. That's not a bad thing. We can learn to rely on God rather than on our own strength. After all, Zechariah 4:6 says that it's not by our might nor by our power, but by God's Spirit.

We need to remember that.

Dreams

What are you hoping to be when you grow up? That's a question we get asked frequently in childhood and early adulthood, but we don't get asked that after we grow up because, well, we've grown up already.

So I have another question. When you became an adult, or when you got your first full-time job that would have been called your vocation, what happened to your dreams? Did they die with that first paycheck? Did they go into hibernation, on the back burner like that project that you always said you were going to do someday?

Remember the excitement of hoping to be something, somebody, and not really knowing how to get there? When you're young, you can have any aspiration and you won't get criticized even though it might not be feasible. Adults smile and nod and pat you on the head and say things like, "Of course you want to be a big red fire engine. Doesn't everybody?"

When I was five years old, I decided I wanted to be a cowboy when I grew up. Shows like Lone Ranger, Gun Smoke, Maverick, and Wild Wild West inspired me. I was going to ride a black horse named Lightning and be able to shoot with the best of them. I'd fall asleep at night dreaming about riding into town and saving the community from the bad guys.

Then I gravitated toward wanting to be a baseball player, then a doctor, and then both. Reality set in at some point, and I had an inclination for law school; then I leaned toward seminary and becoming a minister; and, finally, I realized I loved mathematics, problem-solving, and computers. That's where my mind was when I entered college, and it stuck. I received a B.S. and then an M.S. in Computer Science, and I thoroughly enjoyed developing software for twenty-five years. Now I'm a writer.

My brother, at an early age, wanted to be an airplane when he grew up—not the pilot, the plane itself. He was 17 years old when he realized he couldn't actually do that. His childhood had been quite happy up to that point.

My kids are going through those stages. My oldest daughter Alex is at a university studying piano; her hopes—her dreams—have narrowed sufficiently so that she knows exactly what she wants. When she was five, we had the following conversation.

"Daddy, why do you go to work?"

"To earn money, Alex."

"So you can go to college?"

"I've already been to college."

"Why did you go to college?"

"So that I could get a job."

"Daddy?"

"Yes, Alex?"

"Do I have to go to college? I think I want to just live with you and Mommy."

"Well, if you want a good job, it helps a lot if you go to college first."

"Daddy?"

"Yes, Alex?"

"I think for my job I will stay home and make my bed every day."

It always bothered Alex that she would one day have to leave her mother and father and go start her own life somewhere. Isn't it great that God orchestrates the maturity process so that we can make the right decisions at times when the right decisions need to be made? What if Alex had made the permanent decision when she was five years old to not go to college, or to not seek a job? That would have been fine with her for a year or two, maybe more. But now, when I listen to her playing the piano, I'm sure glad she made the decision she did.

In some ways isn't that analogous to our lives? We think we know exactly what we need; we know exactly what we want. When we ask for it, God turns us down. Why? It's like Alex and making her bed. The right answer for Alex's career plans has nothing to do with making her own bed. She didn't see that when she was five years old, but she saw it later.

Maybe I don't see it at my age, either. God has something planned for me, but I can't see it yet. I can't wait to find out what it is.

My other kids have unique dreams as well. Each wants to make a difference; each wants to be somebody. I hope they never stop dreaming, never stop thinking that someday they can change the world.

As much as I want them to live comfortable lives, I don't want them chasing money. I want them chasing their dreams. Sure, I don't want them living in poverty either, but if they're passionate about what they do, they'll be successful enough to make a living at it.

So here's the catch. Our dreams lead to our plans, but our plans invariably change. God's dreams for us are different than the paths we had intended to take. We need to dream, yes. But we need to dream with the realization that our Creator has plans for us that are wildly different than anything we could imagine.

Once upon a time there was a brilliant young scholar who was a Jewish man rising in the ranks of the elite; then one day on the road to Damascus he had an enlightening experience. He found Christ; well, Christ found him. The man was Saul, who was called Paul after that conversion.

Paul could have been a lawyer, doctor, or anything else he desired. Paul was a tent maker. He could have made big money doing anything, including preaching. Instead, his focus was on something different. He had a message he needed to share. He had dreams that were following something bigger than his own personal desires. Wow! Was he successful! Rich? No, not at all. But successful? You bet.

What do I want to be when I grow up? I still have dreams. I still dream about riding into town on a horse and saving the day. Maybe someday I will.

What do you do when your dream blows up? How do you respond when illness quietly, stealthily dismantles your latest dreams, your aspirations, and your goals? Do you feel cheated; do you go into depression; or do you smile upward and thank God that he apparently has better ideas for you?

Portrait of a Non-Artist as a Young Boy

Our plans are faulty, partly because our perceptions of ourselves—our strengths, our talents, and our needs—can be totally backward at times.

In fourth and fifth grade, I took an art class with Mrs. Hibble and a handful of students on Saturday mornings. On our first day of class, Mrs. Hibble started us with pastels. She asked us to draw an apple that looked so delicious that someone would want to eat it.

I drew a circle—apples are round after all—and a little line for the stem. I was done. But then I looked across the table. Sally was drawing a table for the apple; Jeff was drawing a three dimensional rendition of the apple; and Mike was shading the apple and highlighting part of it. My little circle looked pretty meager at that point.

Mrs. Hibble walked by, asking if we were done. I replied that I had a little bit left. She took one of my pastels and bent down in front of me—I couldn't quite see what she was doing—and when she stood back up I saw that I had a beautiful apple on my sketch pad. I guess my apple looked better than I originally thought. Maybe the light or the angle had thrown me off at first.

At that moment, I had the epiphany that perhaps I might have potential to be a gifted artist.

For the next two years, we did all kinds of artistic works: pastels and water colors, oils and acrylics, short quick projects, and major masterpieces.

Mrs. Hibble obviously thought I had a lot of potential because she spent so much time at my side, saying she was helping me fine tune my work. My art must have been good, I remember thinking, if all it needed was a little touch-up. I figured that the other students in the room just didn't have that knack and that their art wasn't salvageable. After all, Mrs. Hibble didn't help them polish their work.

Usually we painted copies of magazine pictures that Mrs. Hibble gave us. I drew cats, houses, rivers—you name it, I could do it.

One Saturday morning, Mrs. Hibble gave us a new assignment. "I want each of you to choose a subject that is meaningful to you, and for the next three weeks we'll work on that." She didn't require that we tell her what we were painting; she just wanted us to use our creativity and surprise her.

My choice was obvious. I was going to paint a picture of Hank Aaron. He was my idol, my hero. I had memorized any and all meaningful statistics even remotely associated with the slugger; I had read every book about him ever written; and I knew I could paint a picture of him with my eyes closed and both hands tied behind my back. Or something like that.

So I began, and I tackled this assignment like there was no tomorrow. "Mrs. Hibble is going to be so surprised, so proud of me," I thought to myself. I worked diligently; I planned each stroke carefully. Should I make it lifelike and realistic like a Da Vinci? Or should I do something more impressionistic in style, like a Monet? I decided to do a combination of both.

Three weeks later, I was ready. Mrs. Hibble went around to each table, examining our work individually. I knew I'd win something. Was she handing out trophies? Money? Candy? Well, it didn't matter. I knew she'd be surprised.

Finally it was my turn.

There was silence for what seemed like the longest time, and then Mrs. Hibble cleared her throat and began, "Ah, let's see. Don't tell me. You painted a ... is this a moose? And these are his antlers?"

Mrs. Hibble was obviously just kidding and having fun with me.

"No ma'am," I responded politely. "Those aren't antlers. It's a baseball bat. This is Hank Aaron. He's a baseball player."

"Oh I see. But is he, um, standing out in the woods in a flower bed perhaps?"

"No ma'am," I again responded. "He's in a stadium. These are people in the stadium, not flowers."

"I see," said Mrs. Hibble, holding her hand up to her mouth as if to cough. Was that a tear I detected in her eye? And was she shaking? She seemed to be biting her lip, as if she wanted to say something but couldn't.

My work had apparently moved her. I didn't know her to be emotional, really, but she seemed to be so pleased with my magnum opus that perhaps she was weeping with joy. She somehow made it back to her desk, where she burst into laughter. One of the students asked her if she was okay, and she made a comment about remembering some joke she had heard the day before.

Anyway, I was encouraged with her response, and I knew I was well on my way to fame and fortune as an artist. Maybe I could even go off and be a painter and not have to finish grade school!

The following week, Mrs. Hibble came to me and said she had a special project for me. I felt honored. She handed me a picture of a white vase with some red roses, and she very carefully and with great detail explained to me what she wanted.

"This must really be for some special occasion," I thought to myself. I also remember thinking how this would be child's play compared to my previous masterpiece.

In almost no time at all, I had a pretty white vase with red roses in oils on a canvas. I was quite pleased with myself. I still had twenty minutes left, so I decided to be creative and surprise Mrs. Hibble a little.

I opened up a tube of green paint and painstakingly went to work. Fifteen minutes later I had a nice amount of greenery flowing down one side of the vase. I had closed my eyes and envisioned our yard at home, and I felt that I had accurately reproduced the ivy and crabgrass. I very carefully detailed the leaves and grasses, vegetation that looked almost lifelike. I knew Mrs. Hibble would be pleased.

A moment later, she stopped by my table to see how things were going.

"Oh my gosh!" she exclaimed. "Oh no, you spilled your green paint! How did that happen? Here, I'll fix it. What an accident! But never mind, it's fixable."

Before I could say a word, she grabbed my big tube of white paint, poured a large glob onto the canvas, and with a few brush strokes my greenery was gone, just like that. It had vanished. Foliage no more.

It was also at that moment that my mind connected everything … mistaking the baseball bat for antlers … the excruciatingly detailed instructions on what she wanted with the flowers … and it dawned on me that perhaps my perspective of my artistic abilities was not actually aligned with Mrs. Hibble's perspective of my artistic abilities.

I was crushed, floored, an ex-aspiring artist. There was no future of artistic fame slated for me. I would have to finish school after all, unless … unless, of course, a market opened up for paintings featuring moose standing in flower beds, but even I knew that wasn't likely.

This served me well later in life as I came to grip with the realization that my perceptions of my strengths and weaknesses did not always match reality.

On Fishing, Moonshine, and Apollo 13

Our best laid plans—even the little things—can go wrong, and the mundane can end up providing a significant amount of unplanned, unanticipated excitement. Plans going awry might not be fun at the time, but it can provide fodder for great stories down the road.

When I was growing up, Dad and I didn't fish every weekend or even every other weekend, but we fished often enough that some of the details of the trips blur together as I think back on them. One day that I'll always remember clearly, though, was a Saturday morning in mid-April of 1970.

Early in the morning, maybe 5:00am, Dad gently woke me up and said, "Let's go." I knew instantly that he wanted to go fishing. I loved those spurious, unplanned (at least unplanned by me, though Dad had done some preparation) fishing trips. I hopped out of bed, threw on some clothes, and we were out the door within ten minutes. Dad had already loaded the '68 white Olds Cutlass station wagon with our poles and fishing tackle, and the trailer and boat were hooked up and ready to go.

On the way to Kentucky Lake, we listened to the radio. NASA was preparing for the launch of Apollo 13, scheduled to happen later that day. Dad explained to me that we wouldn't be able to fish the whole day because we had company coming that evening, and we needed to get home to help clean the house and prepare dinner. Dad was hoping we would have fresh fish on the menu.

Dad began maneuvering us toward his favorite fishing hole.

"See that cove?" Dad pointed to an open area of shoreline. I nodded. "Let's plan on having lunch there in three or four hours. Mom made sandwiches for us. It'll give us a chance to stretch our legs."

The first half of the morning passed pretty uneventfully. We weren't having much success with the fishing, and after about three hours in the boat Dad steered us over toward the cove for our lunch break.

Dad cut the motor off, not knowing how shallow it might be there, and we drifted in toward the shore. As we got closer, I saw wisps of smoke that seemed to be floating up from the woods not too far away.

"What's that smoke, Dad?" I asked.

As if on cue, a man stepped out from behind a tree, and he had a shotgun in his arms. He wasn't pointing it at us, but he wasn't just casually hanging on to it either. He had a pretty firm grip on that gun.

I only remember two things about the man's appearance. He was wearing overalls, and he looked meaner than any bad guy I had ever seen on TV.

"You boys won't be gettin' out here now, will ya," he said. He wasn't asking a question.

Dad's quick response was, "No, I guess we won't." With deft use of an oar, Dad turned us around and got us back out of that cove almost before I knew what was happening. We decided to eat in the boat. Our lunch plans had been altered, but we sure didn't want to mess with the plans of the guy with the gun.

It wasn't until sometime later that Dad revealed to me that the man was probably moonshining, and he most likely had a still in the woods nearby, making alcohol.

The rest of the morning passed quickly. We caught three fish—a bass and two bullheads—and around noon Dad said it was time to pick up and go. We loaded up the car, got the boat back up on the trailer, and headed home.

We were driving down an old back road—not a highway by any stretch, but a more direct route that Dad knew. Dad turned on the radio and picked up the countdown for the rocket launch.

"Ten!" exclaimed the voice on the radio.

I was excited. Less than a year earlier, I had watched on television (along with the rest of the world) as Neil Armstrong stepped onto the moon.

"Nine!"

I was hoping that Mom and my brother and sister were watching the broadcast back home so that they could tell me about it.

"Eight!"

I was thinking about what it might be like to be an astronaut. I hadn't really considered that as a career. I still wanted to be a professional baseball player, but I figured maybe I could do both.

"Seven!"

I wish we had caught more fish. I guess planning a meal around something not yet caught isn't a great idea.

"Six!"

I thought more about that guy with the shotgun. That was scary.

"Five!"

The tension was building!

"Four!"

I held my breath!

"Three!"

My heart was racing!

BOOM!

The car swerved!

Dad hit the brakes and pulled us to a quick stop. He stepped out of the car, walked around the front, and then he smiled and shook his head. One of our tires had blown out.

Across the road from us was a farmhouse, and a man, woman, and two kids came running out of the house.

"Are you okay?" they asked us. "We were watching the rocket launch and we heard a boom!"

"Yes sir," replied Dad. "Just blew out a tire."

They were relieved, as I'm sure Dad was as well. A flat tire was no fun, but at least it was only a tire and not something worse.

The man told Dad he could pull the car into their driveway, a safer place to change the tire. We laughed about the "boom" and we enjoyed meeting each other as Dad changed the tire. They gave us tall glasses of lemonade. Dad gave them the fish.

As we pulled into our driveway when we reached home, everyone came out to greet us.

My brother and sister were excited. "You missed the rocket! It was cool!" they said.

"Did you bring home enough fish for dinner?" Mom smiled expectantly. "Oh, and how was your lunch?"

Dad just shook his head and laughed.

Time Is Running

As we rounded the turn in one of Schenectady, New York's parks, I drank deeply of the fragrance of the new spring grass that had only recently dared to reach out its fragile fingers, grasping the golden sunlight of that late March Saturday morning. The winter had been a long one—certainly it was the most snow I had seen in my young twenty-five years—and this, our last training run before the half-marathon, was the first without the worries of encountering snow and ice on the sidewalks and streets.

"Almost ... there," I huffed and puffed. "Only two miles to go," I added, breathing hard but enjoying the pace. It was faster than we had been running the past few weeks, and in my racing experience I knew that everything pointed to having a good race the following weekend.

Dan said nothing. Dan usually kept quiet during the runs; he made his statement with his feet and legs rather than any needless verbiage. So I did most of the talking.

Truth be told, I felt more or less obliged to do the talking. After all, I was the one who had talked Dan into signing up for the half-marathon. He had run a lot of 5Ks and 10Ks in his youth. "No, Joel, I'm not going to do a half-marathon," he had emphatically stated.

"No problem," I assured him. "Just come and train with me a little. We'll run some 10Ks."

And we did. We ran together at least a couple of nights each week for several months and on two or three Saturday mornings. That was no small feat, considering the brutal Schenectady winter that still gives me shivers when I think about it. The winter had been a typical one there—not nearly as cold as the Midwest, but we saw at least one ten-inch snowfall per week from December through the middle of March. Most of our training runs found us sloshing through snow and ice. But Dan stuck it out; he showed up to every run we had scheduled.

After each training run, I shared my observations with Dan. He was getting stronger and faster; his endurance was increasing at an admirable rate; and finally he grudgingly agreed to run in the half-marathon. "But only if you do," he declared. I assured him I would be right there by his side.

Now, I should explain that I knew Dan well—after all, we were colleagues at GE's Research and Development Lab in Schenectady. Dan was a talented and gifted individual; he had the Midas touch. He was confident, yet humble; a leader, yet willing to serve; and a brilliant thinker, yet encouraging others to share ideas. In fact, the only area of his life in which he wasn't confident was his running. But honestly, his running was looking good.

The race was scheduled for the first Sunday in April at ten o'clock, starting at the old Proctor Theater downtown. Dan and I agreed to meet at the corner near the theater thirty minutes prior. That would give us sufficient time to warm up and get our nerves settled. It promised to be a big race. Several hundred runners—perhaps even a thousand—had signed up.

I saw Dan at lunch on the Friday before the race. "Don't back out on me now, buddy," I told him. "We've trained too hard for this. Show up or you're dead meat."

Dan laughed and said, "I'll be there."

I opened my eyes that Sunday morning. I looked out the window—crisp sunny blue skies. It looked perfect outside and I was excited. I loved racing.

It was eight o'clock. I had plenty of time, so I made a pot of coffee and a couple of slices of toast. I didn't want to eat anything else until after the race.

Eight twenty. I grabbed a book and sat down to read.

My eyes skimmed the pages but the words remained unread. I wasn't thinking about the book. I was worried that Dan wouldn't show up. Oh, it wasn't that I minded running the race alone. I knew I could do that. I was just worried that Dan would back out, after having trained so hard. I decided to call him.

I picked up the phone and began dialing ... and then I chuckled to myself and put the phone back on the hook. I didn't need to call Dan. He was as reliable as the sun. If there was anybody on this planet who held true to his word, it was Dan. Besides, if he weren't going to show up, he would have called me.

I silently breathed a sigh of relief. Eight forty-five. I hopped off the couch and began doing some light stretching. Nine o'clock. I sat back on the couch and tried to read again, but I couldn't focus on the words.

I leaned back and closed my eyes, visualizing my pace for the race. Back in those days, I ran often enough that I knew what it felt like to run a seven-minute pace (per mile) versus a six forty-five pace versus a six thirty pace. For this half-marathon, Dan and I were targeting a seven-minute pace. We hoped to run the race in just a bit over one and one-half hours.

I opened my eyes. Nine fifteen. It was time for me to go. I drove downtown and parked the car.

Nine twenty-eight. I crossed the street and stood at the corner where Dan and I had agreed to meet. He wasn't there yet.

Nine thirty. Dan still wasn't there. The odd thing, though, was that nobody else was there either. I knew thirty minutes might be a little early, but usually at these races the race officials were there a couple of hours in advance.

Nine thirty-five. Then nine thirty-six. Then nine thirty-seven, thirty-eight, and thirty-nine.

At nine forty, I walked to Proctor Theater, just half a block down from where I had been waiting for Dan. A custodian was sweeping the large canopied shelter in front of the theater. He nodded to me. I nodded to him.

He nodded to me again. I nodded to him again. Then he walked toward me. I figured he was going to tell me I could not loiter in the area.

"You here for the race?" he asked.

"Yes sir," I nodded.

He shook his head and laughed, "They done left."

"Pardon?"

"The race. They done left already."

"What? They started early?"

"I don't know. All I know is 'bout an hour ago, there was a whole bunch of people here. Then somebody said get ready. And somebody said get set. And somebody fired a gun. And all them runners took off."

"They can't do that!" I argued. "They changed the start time for the race? I didn't see any announcement for that. When exactly did it start?"

"Oh, I reckon it started right about ten o'clock."

"But it's only nine fifty now," I said, looking at my watch.

The man laughed again, and then the realization hit me.

Daylight Savings Time!

What was it that Mom had taught me—spring forward, fall back? The spring time change, in those days, always landed on the first Sunday in April.

I had missed the start of the race!

I ran back to my car. I knew what streets were on the race route, so I picked a street parallel to one long stretch of the route and drove in the direction of the race. "Let's see ... Dan will be running at this pace, so at ten o'clock—I mean eleven o'clock—he should be about ... here."

I pulled the car over to the side of the road, one block off the course, and watched runners come by, one at a time. Sure enough, six or seven minutes later, I saw Dan. I waved as he approached. He smiled. I jumped out into the group of runners and stepped into pace alongside my friend.

"Forgot ... the ... time change ... didn't you," he huffed and puffed.

"Yep, sure did," said I, not puffing or huffing. I ran the rest of the race with him, talking and chatting all the way. Dan let me talk. For the last four miles of the race, I apologized.

As I approached the finish line, I did the courteous thing and yelled out, "Bandit," as I stepped aside so that I would not mess up the results.

Dan was a forgiving guy, but he never did run another race with me after that.

You know, we can do all the planning we want. We can even talk others into going along with our plans. We are not infallible. We are human. I, for one, am glad that God's plans supersede mine.

I just hope heaven doesn't have Daylight Savings Time.

On Impeachment

We had a ravine going through the middle of a postage-stamp-sized backyard at the first house my wife and I owned after we married. The fact that several tall trees provided shade near the house meant that any garden or fruit trees would have to be planted on the hill across the ravine.

Our second autumn at that house, we planted a peach tree on the hill. We tended it and nurtured it, and that tree got off to a good start in life. My wife loved that peach tree. Over time, though, some weeds and small saplings grew up on the hill as well: small pine trees, tulip poplars, mimosas, and sweet gums.

Fast forward two and a half years. My wife went away for the weekend, leaving me with a list of things she wanted me to think about doing. It didn't surprise me to see "weed and chop down trees on the hill" on the list, and in parentheses was written the remark, "don't chop down the peach tree." My wife must have chuckled when she wrote that rather obvious note, knowing I would chuckle too.

I started the task of taking out the saplings. I've always enjoyed that kind of mindless task where I can sing songs or think about things while I'm moving in a rhythm, a pattern of steps leading to some final accomplishment. Also, I've always enjoyed being outside. With this project, then, I had the best of both worlds. I don't recall what song I might have been singing, though likely it was my favorite outdoor yard work song, "Give Me Oil in My Lamp." My sister, brother, and I used to sing that song for hours while, as kids, we weeded the front walk or pulled dandelions or chopped down mimosas.

Anyway, back to the saplings on the hill ... there I was, singing and chopping, chopping and singing, pleased that I was outside and doubly pleased that I, once again, was participating in a man-versus-nature battle.

This felt like a piece of cake. I'd chop down a sapling, take a step to my right, chop down another sapling, take a step to my right, and that's how it went.

"Give me oil in my lamp, keep me burning, give me oil in my lamp, I pray (hallelujah!)." Chop ... step ... chop ... step.

When I reached the other end of the hill, I stood up and scanned my progress. I had gotten every sapling on the hill along with most of the weeds too. I was done!

"Don't chop down the peach tree!"

Those words suddenly appeared out of nowhere, kind of like how the voice of God speaks to Noah in the old Bill Cosby skit.

"Who said that?"

It was my conscience, perhaps—I'm not sure—but at any rate, I had a sinking feeling in my stomach that my plans for the day had just changed.

I scanned the hill again, hoping beyond hope that I hadn't really done what I was quickly realizing I had indeed done.

Ouch.

Peach tree, no more. There was none in sight. I had chopped down the peach tree.

I checked my watch. My wife was scheduled to come back that afternoon. I had four hours to attempt to remedy the situation. I got on the phone and started calling area nurseries.

"Sorry Bud, we're out of peach trees."

"Nope, just sold the last one," said another.

A third nursery informed me, "Our peach trees arrive on Wednesday. Call back then."

The search continued until I finally found a small local nursery that said they had peach trees remaining. I hopped in the car and drove there as quickly as I could.

Their selection of peach trees comprised one meager little stick that had a remarkable resemblance to the Charlie Brown Christmas tree in that television special. If I had put an ornament on top, the tree would have bent over to the ground.

I looked at my watch and discovered I only had about two hours left.

"I'll take it!" I exclaimed enthusiastically, to the astonishment of the store clerk.

"You will?" he exclaimed. "You're not going to ask for a discount or something?"

I didn't have time to barter.

"Nope, I'll take it. Gotta go. Thanks."

I raced home, grabbed a shovel, and in about thirty minutes I had the tree sitting nicely in approximately the same spot where its predecessor had enjoyed its short life in our backyard.

When my wife arrived home, I explained what had happened. I knew that being up front and honest—and demonstrating that I had thoughtfully provided a replacement tree—was the only thing to do, and I knew that my loving and caring and forgiving spouse would be, well, loving and caring and forgiving.

Of course she was. I only had to sleep on the couch downstairs for a couple of months.

All right, it wasn't that bad. It would have been better though if the tree had survived. It didn't. Within six months it was dead, gone, ceasing to exist.

At any rate, this whole saga intensely heightened my appreciation for great peaches, and I love them now more than ever. It also reminded me that things don't always go according to our plans. Sometimes we just have to improvise and keep going.

God's Plans

Planning—the ability to think ahead and make appropriate preparations—is not strictly limited to humans. Even squirrels have the innate sense to bury nuts in the ground for winter. Being able to plan beyond the basic food and safety requirements, though, might be uniquely a homo sapiens trait. We plan for education; we plan for careers; we plan for retirement; and we even plan where our belongings go when we die, should we end up with excess.

We even try to plan to account for catastrophes and other unplanned events. We take out home and auto insurance policies, disability insurance policies, long-term care insurance policies, etc., in an attempt to be ready for the unexpected.

The plans that we cast for ourselves are not necessarily the same as God's plans for us. First of all, let's get something clear. God knows us, inside and out—after all, he made us—and he also knows our futures. That is, God knows how the days are mapped out for each of us, from beginning to end.

The thing is, God wants us to depend on him. God wants us to experience his lavish love for us first hand. I'm not saying that preparation is bad. I'm saying that you shouldn't be too surprised when all your careful planning starts unraveling.

Chronic illness can rip apart your plans in a heartbeat.

Art from the European Renaissance was often expressed in tapestries illustrating several events; for example, different milestones in a king's life. In some sense, God sees our lives like that. He can see everything that's going to happen.

> All the days ordained for me were written
> in your book before one of them came to be.
>
> —Psalm 139:16b

Not only does he know what's going to happen to each of us, but he has a purpose for each of us as well.

> The Lord will fulfill his purpose for me;
> your love, O Lord, endures forever—
> do not abandon the works of your hands.
>
> —Psalm 138:8

Note that the question isn't, "What's my purpose in life?" The question is really, "What's God's purpose for me?"

I don't believe for one second that God just sits idly by, watching a day's events unfold without ever intervening. It's also obvious, though, that God doesn't rescue us from every possible harm. He allows us to make mistakes; he allows misfortune to happen; and sometimes he calls us home before (from our perspectives) we're good and ready.

Why is that? I don't know. I do know that I'm glad he has a plan for my life and that he is going to see it through. If I had to depend on my own strength to carry out my life's work, I'd be in big trouble. He allows our plans to get frustrated, and (if we look) we can see him constantly working in our lives.

IV

The Prayer Relationship

We have to pray with our eyes on God,
not on the difficulties.

Oswald Chambers

March 12, 2010

I was 10 years old when I started following Nebraska football. We won the National Championship that year. That was Nebraska's second consecutive championship, but I hadn't noticed the first one just the year before. We bought our first color television set the night before the bowl game at the end of that '71 season, anticipating a great game between the undefeated Huskers and Bear Bryant's undefeated Crimson Tide of the U. of Alabama. It was supposed to be a blow-out— sports writers all over were predicting Nebraska would be decimated by the Tide. Well, it was a blow-out indeed, only it went the other way. Nebraska won, 38–6.

For years after that, Husker fans waited in anticipation of the next championship. Year after year, we came close. We "almost" won in 1982, when a horrible officiating call ended up giving Penn State a win, our only loss of the season. In the 1984 Orange Bowl, we lost in a heart-breaker to Miami (I was at that game, my last in the marching band). In the 1994 Orange Bowl, we lost on a last second field goal to Florida State. We just couldn't seem to pull out the big win when it mattered.

But then ... we beat Miami in the '95 Orange Bowl to win the championship ... and we beat (destroyed) Florida in the '96 Fiesta Bowl to win the championship again ... and then we crushed Tennessee in the '98 Orange Bowl to win again, the third time in four years.

Those were giddy times. During my oldest son's first five years on this planet, the Huskers were 60–3. That's pretty impressive.

Looking back, I can say it was worth the wait.

There's an old adage that says the good things in life are worth waiting for.

Even with the preposition at the end of that sentence, it's probably true.

There are things I want in life. I want another championship.

I want to see my kids succeed in life, by whatever definition of success is the most meaningful.

I want to be done with Parkinson's Disease, once and for all.

So, a week and three days after surgery, I'm sitting here. My hands ache from typing; I'm stuttering this morning as usual; I'm shuffling when I walk, and I'm waiting for my medicine to kick in.

But what about the surgery? This thing I had done—the injecting of the virus—is going to take time, if it works at all. I want to get better so that I can play with my kids (well, I do play with them, but I want to run at full speed in the back yard all the time, not just some of the time) ... I want (someday) to play with grandkids. I don't want them to remember their grandpa as some old guy who couldn't walk and who drooled.

Anyway, I'm waiting for another championship, a victory over Parkinson's. That might be the sweetest championship of all, this side of heaven.

On the other hand ... when I look at all the people who have recently been praying for me, I see this huge cloud of witnesses. People everywhere are pulling for me, praying for me, and encouraging me. Hardly a day goes by without someone saying, "Hey, we're thinking about you." I feel sort of like the Olympic performer who finished his event and then went to the sidelines, waiting for the judges' scores. I'm hoping for a string of 10's, or 9.8's or something. Who knows. Maybe it'll end up as a string of 0's. But we tried.

Will it work? Dunno. God has provided a peace about the whole thing. He's telling me to keep moving forward. Don't look back and wait.

I'm excited though ... I'm terribly excited. I feel like a kid waiting for Christmas to come.

Hide and Seek with Mom

We lived in Clarksville, Tennessee for a while in my childhood, and during that time Dad would come home from work every day at 6pm in his little red Opal. He would turn off the main road, Madison Street, into our pastoral subdivision, and sometimes Mom would walk with us kids to meet him on the road. We would shout with excitement when we could see his car in the traffic.

On one snowy evening, Dad called and said he'd be a little late. We all—including Mom—wanted to go walking in the snow anyway, so we put on our coats, stocking caps, and gloves, and we ventured out into the crisp night air. The snow was still falling gently and there was no wind that evening, so it was quite a pleasant walk as we crunched, crunched, crunched down the road.

When we reached the edge of the subdivision, we turned around and headed toward home. Mom said, "Let's play hide and seek! I'll hide first." We kids very dutifully closed our eyes and counted to 50, and then the search began.

It was snowing a little harder and we couldn't see too far ahead, but I had read enough of the Hardy Boys to know that all we really needed to do was to follow Mom's footprints in the snow. It was a little tough because we were walking over the tracks we had made coming out, but with the snowfall Mom's latest steps were relatively easy to follow.

"Look!" my little brother exclaimed when we reached our driveway, as he pointed to the left. The tracks veered off into the woods. Anticipating that we'd find Mom at any moment, we quickened our pace and followed the steps into the woods. I remember thinking I'd have to talk to Mom about how to cover her footprints, sweeping them with a branch or something so that they'd be harder to see.

At any rate, we marched and marched and marched and—suddenly the tracks stopped. Right there, at the base of a fairly large tree, the trail of Mom's footprints ended.

"Where'd she go?" my sister asked.

I whistled, impressed. "Mom must have figured out that she needed to cover her tracks," I said. We circled the tree, but she had done a great job hiding her footsteps. We each decided to go a different direction—Jen to the left, Barry to the right, and I straight.

We assigned signals so that we could communicate: Jen was an owl and would do a "hoot hoot" call; Barry was a bobwhite and would do the "bob white, bob white" whistle; and I, of course, was the coyote with a ferocious "A-Woooooooo" howl.

We took our respective paths deeper into the woods. I was thoroughly enjoying this adventure. I had fully expected to find Mom in another minute or two. But ... three or four minutes passed, then five, and still no sign of our female parental unit.

Then I heard, "Bob white, bob white."

I answered back with a hearty "A-Wooooooo," and I heard Jennie respond with her "hoot hoot" off in the distance.

The sounds of the bobwhite repeated.

I wondered if Barry had found her. I started walking back towards him, following my tracks. It was then that I realized that even though we had assigned our animal call signals, we hadn't said what the signals meant. The "bob white, bob white" could have meant that he found Mom, but it could have meant any number of things.

"Did you find her?" I asked excitedly when I was within talking range. Jennie joined us at the same time.

"No," said Barry, "but I have to go to the bathroom. Can we go home now?"

"Well, I guess so," I said, disappointed at not having found Mom.

So the three of us started heading home. After two or three steps, though, Jen said, "Hey wait, we can't leave Mom out here."

"Oh yeah," we agreed in unison. We called out, "Mom! Mom! Ma-aaaaaaaaaam!"

Nothing.

We called again. No response. We walked around the woods for another minute or two, ending up very near to where Mom's tracks had ended at the base of the tree.

There was silence for a moment or two, and then ... a laugh warmed the snow-filled darkness.

Where was she? I didn't see her in front of us, nor was she to the left or to the right. Spinning around, I expected to see Mom there.

Nothing.

Then Jen said, "Hey, look!" and she pointed up in the tree. Above us, perhaps fifteen feet off the ground, sat a bundled figure barely discernible in the darkness.

"Mom!" I exclaimed. "How did you get up there?"

She climbed down, laughing, and we all joined in the laughter as we hiked back to the house, looking forward to a warm meal and some hot chocolate and marshmallows.

Years later, though the story has grown foggy and some of the details have been embellished with time, a key point is not lost on me. When searching and seeking answers, look up. There is one Truth, and he is God.

Are you walking through life, eyes downward, following tracks that lead nowhere? Look up.

Squeaky Bottom No More

I've never been particularly handy around the home, but I haven't let that lack of ability stop me from breaking things as I try to fix something else.

At least I try. Dad always told me, "Don't just stand there; do something, even if it's wrong." I'm also trying to instill that "try hard" ethic in my kids, so when opportunities come up at home to fix or repair something I try to involve one or more of the kids so they can use it as a learning opportunity.

A few years ago, our water heater started acting up. It would still heat the water, but it was slow and the water wasn't getting all that hot. It seemed like one of the two heating elements wasn't working. I went to the hardware store, found a matching element, and took it home.

My oldest son Nathan and I went into the crawl space underneath the house to look at the water heater. I had the right-sized wrench with me. After struggling with the heating element for ten minutes, I acknowledged I was having trouble removing it. I decided that part of the element may have partially rusted onto the body of the water tank, so I decided to go get some WD–40 to see if I could loosen it.

I left and returned a minute later.

I sprayed the WD–40 and set the can down. I waited a minute or two, and Nathan and I chatted about random things. I picked up the wrench and tried again to turn the element. Nothing.

Then I decided to get serious, so I put my whole body into it, bending my knees and putting as much of my weight on that wrench as I could. Suddenly I heard a "Shhhhhhhh" sound.

"Nathan, did you hear that? I think we have a leak somewhere."

"Dad—"

"Son, I'm going to pull down on this wrench again. Listen for the sound."

"Shhhhhh," the sound repeated.

"Yep, we've got a leak, Son."

"Dad—"

"I wonder if it's a leak in the drain valve."

"Dad—"

"I hope it's not a leak in the base."

"Dad—"

"What is it Son?"

"When you kneel, you're sitting on the can of WD–40. The spray is what's making the noise."

I reached back and felt my bottom.

Nathan was right.

My bottom didn't squeak for months after that.

Why do I get so stuck on my own thoughts, so determined to do things my way, that I fail to listen to others who may have better ideas? That affects my prayer life too. How often does my own refusal to listen cause me to miss what God is trying to tell me?

> Trust in the Lord with all your heart
> and lean not on your own understanding;
> in all your ways acknowledge him,
> and he will make your paths straight.
> —Proverbs 3:5–6

The Witch

Many years ago I was one of a group of four adults who took turns teaching a Sunday School class for three-year-olds. Now, on one particular Sunday, we had invited parents to come join us so they could see first-hand how we ran the class and what kinds of things we were teaching. Our little cadre of teachers was proud of how we kept the class very Bible-based, reading stories from the Bible each week.

For the previous week's lesson we learned about Lydia, a woman who sold purple cloth to rich customers.

In the class, I asked the kids, "Whom did we talk about last week?"

One girl raised her hand and shouted out, "Lydia!"

"Very good," I responded, proud that my obviously effective teaching methods were having an impact on the kids. "And who can tell me about Lydia," I continued.

Another kid raised his hand and answered, "Lydia sold purple cloth."

Again I responded with, "Very good," probably praising myself more than I was actually praising the child who answered.

So I kept going. "Who remembers who bought Lydia's purple cloth?"

There was silence for a moment, and then one boy raised his hand and said, "The witch!"

I was horrified. The witch? We hadn't talked about a witch. I certainly didn't want the parents getting the wrong idea about the content of our discussions in class. The class was taking a different direction than I had intended.

"The witch?" I meekly asked.

"Yes," he affirmed. "The witch."

There was a pause for what was probably less than a second but felt like an eternity. Then the boy continued. "The witch," he said again. "Weally, weally witch people."

You know, not only do we worry too much, but we tend to try to orchestrate everything to a tee. We want perfection. That's not how life works, though, at least not on this side of heaven. God wants us to depend on him. It is okay for your direction to change when God is the one steering. Sure, we need to prepare, but I wonder how often a Sunday school class goes awry because the teacher has spent too much time preparing a fancy lesson and not enough time in prayer. God knows what's in our hearts; he knows our needs better than we do. He would like us to get to know him as well as he knows us.

He Knows Your Name

Back in my carefree days of only three kids, there was a period where I would try to take one kid out for breakfast each week. Sometimes we'd go to the Riz Raz Cafe, where the waitresses always greeted me with a yell across the room—"Mornin' Honey"—or sometimes we'd go to a local coffee shop.

Nathan, when he was six or seven, especially enjoyed going to the coffee shop and ordering a vanilla steamer, though sometimes he'd be adventurous and get a raspberry steamer. The guy behind the counter became friends of sorts with Nathan and always called him "Bud."

The guy—his name was Gus—would see Nathan and would ask, "Vanilla steamer, Bud?" and Nathan would nod and break out in a big smile. Gus would always deliver a perfect vanilla steamer with extra foam to Nathan. I'm not sure why Gus called Nathan "Bud," except that I think Gus probably called just about everybody that.

It came to pass that one morning for whatever reason we decided to go to a different coffee house. We walked in, and Nathan approached the counter cautiously. At his young age, he wasn't one to embrace change easily.

I placed my order and then it was Nathan's turn. He looked up at me, and I bent down and whispered in his ear, "Do you want a vanilla steamer?" Nathan nodded. I then told him to tell that to the man behind the counter.

Nathan did just as I asked.

The man leaned over the counter and said, "One vanilla steamer coming right up, Bud."

Nathan's eyes opened wide in astonishment.

In a couple of minutes our drinks were ready, and we sat down at a table. I could tell something was bothering Nathan.

We said a prayer over our breakfast, and then Nathan looked and asked, "Daddy?"

"Yes?" I replied.

"How did that man know my name?"

You know, wouldn't it be neat if everyone really knew your name? I'm always amazed when I'm sitting at a traffic intersection and I look around at the people in the surrounding cars and I discover that I don't know anybody. Numerous times I've told my kids that I'm astonished at how many people in this world I don't know.

It feels almost as though we should have weekly gatherings—maybe even daily—so that strangers can become friends.

But we know one thing for certain. There is someone who really does know all of our names. He knows the number of hairs on our heads (or in my case the number that I used to have). He knows all our sorrows and worries and concerns; he also knows our joys and victories and dreams.

He cares about you. Someday when you come face to face with him, he won't call you Bud (unless that's your name). He will call you by your real name. He will look you in the eyes and he will look you in the heart.

That will be even better than getting a perfect vanilla steamer with extra foam from Gus.

A Golden What?

We do not always communicate effectively. We use the wrong words; we misunderstand what is said to us; and we twist words (or remain silent) to keep out of trouble. The following anecdotes illustrate these points.

The kids and I were driving through town on our way to church one Sunday afternoon, and my oldest daughter Alex, who was six at the time, saw a beautiful large, yellow dog standing on the sidewalk next to the road. Alex said, "That dog is so pretty! I think it's a Golden ... I think it's a Golden Delicious."

My kids all love to read, and occasionally comical situations will arise when they mispronounce words they have never heard spoken. One day, youngest son Aaron and I were fishing in a canoe. Out of the blue, Aaron asked, "How much does a *yakd* cost?"

"A yakd?" I asked.

"Yes," he affirmed, "a yakd."

"Ummm, what's a yakd?" I asked.

He responded, "You know, those big, fancy boats like the ones we saw in the harbor this morning."

It took me just a moment to realize that he meant yacht. I was laughing so hard I almost fell out of the canoe.

"How did you sleep?" Grandma asked five-year old Nathan, my oldest son, at breakfast.

Nathan stared at her, trying to figure out why she would ask that question. Finally, he put his hands together, placed them up against his cheek, put his head down on the table, and said, "Like this."

Four-year old Laura was alone in her room with the door closed, which was unusual for her. I knocked on the door and asked, "Laura, are you okay?"

After a few seconds of silence, I heard a meek voice answer, "Yes."

Not convinced, I knocked on the door. "May I come in?"

A few moments later, the doorknob turned and the door opened. Laura, hands behind her back, stood by the door and looked up at me. Her lips, chin, and cheeks were covered in chocolate. "Have you been eating anything?" I asked.

She looked surprised that I would even remotely suspect such a thing, and she said, "Mmmmm, uh, no."

I told her, "Well that's good, because you know you're not supposed to eat in your room, and if you DO eat in your room then I might not let you have chocolate ever again for the rest of your life." Since then, she's either kept it very secret or she's been very obedient. I'm not sure which.

God not only knows what we mean, but he knows what we're going to say before we say it. Not only that, but God knows what we need even better than we do. That's reassuring to me. Don't worry about getting the words right. What he really wants is for you to spend time with him.

Prayer and Your Relationship with God

I've read that any person on earth is at most five handshakes away from any other person. That almost boggles the mind. Who is the most famous person with whom you have shaken hands? Who is the most famous person with whom you are just two handshakes away?

If you could pick anybody, past or present, to talk to for an hour, asking any questions you want, whom would you choose?

Would you choose a president or CEO? Would you pick a famous athlete or movie star?

What would you say if I told you that every day you have an opportunity to sit down with the King of kings, the Lord of lords?

Well, you do.

God is the source of our wisdom; God is the source of our inspiration; God is the source of our strength and our salvation. He is the creator, the redeemer, and the most trustworthy friend you can imagine.

Every morning upon awakening, you have the opportunity to say hello to the most powerful figure in the whole universe. You can talk his ears off or you can sit and listen. Preferably you would do some of both. He likes listening to you. Even though he knows what you're going to say, when you tell him about your fears, your concerns, and your needs, it's his way of off-loading the worries to him so that you can end up with a smile on your face.

So ... why haven't I been healed yet?

There is debate about how God answers prayer. Some of it stems from Matthew 7:7, where we read:

Ask and it will be given to you; seek and you will find; knock and the door will be opened to you.

—Matthew 7:7

I've heard people argue that this means you can ask for anything you want, and God will give it to you. Then people chime in with this: "I've asked for things that I haven't received. Does that mean this passage is not true?" Others may respond with, "Well, God answers prayers with 'no' sometimes." Still others argue that God doesn't say no, but that unanswered prayer is simply a "not yet."

Hold everything. The problem with all of this is that we're trying to make God fit a pattern. We're acting like magicians trying to get the incantation just right, thinking that if we say the right things then God will answer and give us what we want.

Prayer isn't a formula. Prayer isn't a magical spell. Prayer is a relationship between the person doing the praying and God. We spend time in prayer so that we can listen to God and talk to God. It's not about bringing our laundry list of things we want. It's about us caring enough about him that we spend time with him.

Think about your relationships with your kids or with your parents. Any parent of a teenager has (I hope) said, "Hey, let me know if you need anything," or, "Let me know if there's anything I can do to help."

That does not mean that we will fulfill our teenager's request to destroy the math teacher before tomorrow morning's test or that we will grant his wish for a million dollars because he doesn't want to enter the work force. We wouldn't do those things, of course.

If the relationship between parent and child is a good one, then the child should be able to approach the parent and say, "Dad, I'm struggling with something ... can you help me?" That's what it's all about.

Yes, God does work miracles. He heals; he gives us the ability to forgive; he gives us peace and joy in times of trial. God wants to be present and active in our lives. We need to make ourselves available to work on that relationship. We are blessed that our creator and our savior also wants to be our best friend, not "the man behind the curtain."

> I am the good shepherd; I know my sheep and my sheep know me—just as the Father knows me and I know the Father—and I lay down my life for the sheep.
>
> —John 10:14–15

It takes time to develop any relationship, and it involves both talking and listening. God already knows you, and he wants you to know him. Are you giving him quality time? Are you giving him your best? Or do you treat God as though he is your little genie in a bottle, your "Open Only in Cases of Emergency" box?

When you pray, are you talking to God or are you really just talking to yourself? Are you listening to God or are you focused only on your desires? I tell you, it's easy to get distracted ... it's easy to think we're listening to the right things, when we're not.

Have you ever been in a noisy, crowded room and heard someone say your name, even though it was only spoken at normal volume? You want to be able to hear God, even in the din and chaos of everyday life. He's waiting for you. Get to know his voice.

V

Peace, Joy, and Courage

Expect great things from God,
attempt great things for God.

William Carey

March 17, 2010

The stitches came out today—March 17th—and it looks as though the incisions are healing nicely. The checkup at Duke was fine—I was "on" as far as medication goes, and my body performed the usual tests the usual ways. I was given the green light for exercise, so now I'll slowly be working my way back into shape.

(I should explain here that when the medicine is effectively working in relieving symptoms, this is called the "on" state in Parkinson's Disease lingo. When the medicine is not working, this is called "off." Being "off" is awful: my body doesn't move well; I feel groggy and lethargic; and my brain doesn't think clearly.)

As of this date, it's way too early to be able to report any improvement. It's going to take months, perhaps a year, in order to say anything has changed. So we'll have to wait and see.

A couple of things have surfaced the past few days, and I don't know that they're surgery-related but they probably are.

First, I've been singing in my sleep for the past several nights—not lyrics, just humming—but I've awakened with happy thoughts and cheerful melodies. My wife is happy ... it sure beats the screaming from nightmares that has been happening off and on for the past several years.

The other thing that has become apparent is that my dyskinesia is much more pronounced than it was. This is the involuntary jerking, twitching, rocking, and swaying that occurs in advanced Parkinson's Disease when too much dopamine is present in the brain. When I'm standing, it looks as if I'm trying to dance without moving my feet (almost like watching Elvis on television in the late 60s).

So ... my eyes blink; my face, neck, and shoulders twitch; I can't sit still (and type); and I can't stand still. It's a feeling that's very similar to being hyper-antsy about something.

Imagine waking up in the morning, drinking a dozen cups of coffee and then a 6-pack of Coke while eating an entire basket of Easter candy, and, well, you'll come pretty close to what dyskinesia feels like. Or maybe not ...

Anyway, I'm not sure if this increase in dyskinesia is a good thing or bad thing ... it can happen when your body gets too much dopamine ... but the surgery isn't really supposed to be supplying more dopamine this quickly.

One of the possible side effects of the surgery was increased dyskinesia, and that may be what's happening. That's still okay ... it doesn't necessarily mean it'll get worse. It's just something for which I need to figure out how to compensate...changing my medicinal regimen over time or something.

But, until the docs say to change, I have to stay on schedule, because only then will we be able to see the effects of the surgery.

Anyway ... we worked out in the garden all afternoon, played football in the backyard after dinner tonight, and I have an 8am tennis match tomorrow morning with a friend from church.

Physically, I'll be able to get back to where I was before surgery, and then we'll wait for the results. Cognitively? We have no idea.

I've had several instances of short term memory lapses the past two weeks ... and it's the weirdest thing. My memory has been excellent all along, so to suddenly not remember something just feels strange.

I'm hoping that's just a short-term side effect of the surgery and it'll go away soon. We'll see.

At any rate, I'm feeling a remarkable sense of peace about this whole thing. God is in control. The peace I felt before and during the experience of surgery has continued in the trenches of the battles of life, even when things seem different than I was hoping.

I am praying for healing, but I am also reminded of what Paul wrote about the "thorn in his flesh."

> Three times I pleaded with the Lord to take it away from me. But he said to me, "My grace is sufficient for you, for my power is made perfect in weakness."

Therefore I will boast all the more gladly about my weaknesses, so that Christ's power may rest on me. That is why, for Christ's sake, I delight in weaknesses, in insults, in hardships, in persecutions, in difficulties. For when I am weak, then I am strong.

—2 Corinthians 12:8–10

Warning: Detour Ahead

The first sign that something was wrong showed up in 1996, at work. I had just been handed a small team of software developers to tackle an emergency project, tasked with adding some security functionality to our operating system software. I scheduled a planning meeting for that afternoon.

I prepared that morning for the meeting, and by the time lunch rolled around I felt ready and confident. This would be a good project; I was confident that the team would be up to the challenge. I decided to go out for my usual lunch-time run. It was hot outside—I loved running in the Carolina heat—and the temperature probably hovered around 95°F on that July day.

After six miles of trails and pavement through Research Triangle Park, I took a quick shower, ate the sandwich I had brought from home, and did final preparations for the meeting.

The meeting started. I was standing at the white board, ready to explain what needed to be done. I opened my mouth, but no words came out.

I coughed and cleared my throat.

Again, no words came out. With some degree of effort, I eventually was able to stammer a few words together, but it was a painful experience for me as a speaker and I know that it was painful for my audience.

In almost no time, I went from being a confident speaker to being a stutterer. I couldn't figure it out. Had I suffered a stroke? After all, I tended to run hard on those hot North Carolina summer days. The run on that particular day had felt good though, and nothing else seemed to indicate that a stroke had occurred.

I eventually talked myself into thinking that it was merely due to stress, just the price one had to pay for climbing the corporate ladder.

As time went on, my speaking slowly grew worse. Then, one evening in the spring of 1998 when I was pouring water into the dinner glasses before sitting down to eat, my daughter asked me, "Daddy, why is your hand shaking?"

I looked down. Sure enough, my hand was shaking. I hadn't noticed it before. I didn't have an answer to the question, other than perhaps it too was because of stress.

Later that fall, I came home late from work one night and found my wife, pregnant with our fourth child, lying in bed and reading a book on Parkinson's Disease. I had almost forgotten anything I knew about that topic, other than the fact that Grandma had died from related complications. My wife had never mentioned the disease. Why would she be reading a book on it?

I asked her bluntly, "Who has Parkinson's Disease?"

She looked up at me with moist eyes and said, "I think you do."

I went into immediate denial.

"Me? Parkinson's is an old person's disease. My grandma had it."

"I know. Remember when we watched home movies at your parents' house during the summer?"

"Yes?"

"There was a video where your grandmother was sitting on the couch. She had no smile."

"I remember that."

"That's what you look like."

"What? I smile."

"You don't smile like you used to."

"I'm still happy inside," I insisted.

"But you don't smile like you used to," she repeated. "Your face doesn't show emotion. There's something called the Parkinson's mask, according to this book. That, and some other things, are making me think you might have Parkinson's."

"What else?"

"You don't swing your left arm when you walk. You shuffle your feet. Your speech is slurred—yes, stuttering can be a symptom of Parkinson's. You're more tired than you used to be."

"I'm only 38. I can't have Parkinson's."

"It says here that 8 to 10 percent of Parkinson's people are under the age of 40. It's called Young Onset Parkinson's Disease or YOPD."

"Really?"

She nodded.

Either I didn't believe it, or I just didn't want to believe it. Looking back, I'm not sure which was the case. At any rate, I had entered a period of denial.

The Diagnosis

My denial continued for several months. We had our fourth child, moved into another house, and I continued the climb up the corporate ladder. I was still hearing comments like "way to go," "atta boy," and "nice work."

However, I was also hearing comments from people who were asking what was wrong with my arm (because it wasn't swinging), what was wrong with my legs (because my feet were shuffling), and what was wrong, period (because my face was frozen in a mask-like appearance). In addition, my speech got worse.

I finally began accepting the fact that my wife might be right. Though I didn't want to be told that I had Parkinson's Disease (or anything else), I knew that something was physically wrong and I wanted to find out its name. I wanted to know the name of the enemy. I decided to go to the family physician.

"It might be essential tremor," he said, "so let's do an experiment. I want you to drink two glasses of red wine every night for a month to see if that changes anything."

That was one of the most relaxing months of my life, but no, it didn't change anything. My doctor scheduled an appointment with a neurologist in Durham, and on September 13, 1999, I met with the neurologist in his clinic. He performed a series of tests and had me stand up and walk and sit down and do all sorts of other basic things. The problem with PD is that there's not a way to diagnose it other than through observation of the symptoms.

After the battery of tests, the neurologist left Michelle and me alone for a few minutes. The room was quiet. I was pretty sure by that point that I had PD. In fact, I knew that it would help to have a name attached to whatever it was making its marks on my body. If I were told that I didn't have PD, I would be back at square one, with no clue what to do next.

When the neurologist returned with his head down, his body language said it all. He sat down, rubbed his hands through his hair, and said softly, "Mr. Schnoor, I'm afraid you have Parkinson's Disease."

I have to tell you right now that when he told me the news, I was filled with an overwhelming sense of peace that I wasn't expecting. There was no "survival instinct" that clicked on; there was no feeling of "okay, take a deep breath, relax, and think this through." I simply felt an assurance that God was there. In fact, I felt so at peace that it caught me off guard. I was relaxed and totally at ease. That's something only God can do.

At that instant, I knew the answer to why my grandmother had been able to have such a sense of peace and joy about her even during her trials with PD. The answer was (and is) that the peace comes from God entirely. It's not something the recipient does, other than trust.

The neurologist urged me to get a second opinion. He also wanted me to have an MRI, just to confirm that what we were seeing was not something caused by a brain tumor.

Incidentally, the MRI was an interesting experience. I kept thinking back to the Stephen Wright quip, "I had an MRI done to see if I was claustrophobic." I was not.

One thing the neurologist said that stuck with me was that on average I could probably expect to have ten to fifteen years of reasonable bodily movement on medications.

Anyway, with the diagnosis there was a sense of relief in knowing what it was that we were fighting. We knew the enemy. I felt God holding me in his hands and saying, "Joel, I'm with you every step of the way."

Nothing compares with the peace God gives us when the world says it's time to panic.

Peace

Nobody plans on being diagnosed with a chronic illness. It's not like the monster under the bed or the shadow in the closet that caused you to shudder at night in your childhood. That is, most people don't live in fear of contracting a chronic illness. Rather, it's something that catches you off-guard.

Parkinson's Disease isn't a physical nuisance. It's a life-changing intruder. It's one thing to go to a theater and to be told, "Sorry Mister, the movie has been canceled tonight." It's something else to be told, "Sorry Mister, we are taking your job away; your plans for retirement have been axed; you won't be doing your favorite hobbies; and we are going to eat away at your life savings faster than termites in a saw mill."

Imagine this scene ...

Ring! Ring! Ring!

I walk to the front door and open it. Standing there is a large man in a circa 1970 leisure suit with a suitcase in one arm and a tuba in the other.

"Hi Joel! I'm your long lost cousin Leoj, and I'm moving in with you," he says only a moment before barging through the doorway.

"I, uh," I stammer, "Hold on a moment. I'll be right back."

I run upstairs to find my wife. Surely she knows about this. Leoj follows me up the stairs.

"Honey, this is Leoj, and he's moving in with us."

"But he can't! We have plans; we have things to do; we have—" argues my wife.

"I'm here, I'm here, I'm here," interrupts Leoj, looking me in the eye, "so get used to it. I will follow you all the days of your life. I will deplete your savings; you'll have to quit your job to take care of me; no more fancy retirement plans for you, Bub. I should warn you that

I practice the tuba day and night. You won't be seeing much sleep. So, get used to it. Now, do you have any pastrami in the fridge? I haven't eaten since Tuesday and I'm starving."

This humorous depiction is not meant to make light of chronic illness, but it does portray the suddenness with which an illness can appear. Instantly, your life is forever changed. How do you respond? Where do you find peace? I guess it depends whether you've built your house on sand or on solid rock.

First, we need to distinguish between the peace that God provides and peace as the world sees it. There is a human peace that we can attempt to get—or to convince ourselves of—when we know we've taken care of whatever needs to be done. For example, when we pay off our credit card debt, we may feel a peace from not having to worry about that part of our financial responsibilities for the time being. That's a human-invoked peace.

The peace that comes from God is not something you can talk yourself into; it's not a trick of the mind; it's not succumbing to apathy or a state of numbness; it's not a mental toughness that you develop over time; and it's not something you can really plan and anticipate.

It is pure, instant, undeserved, amazing, total, unexpected, and complete, and it comes at exactly the right time and in exactly the right amount.

In other words, it is perfect. Are you surprised?

Peace is one of the fruits of the Spirit that Paul lists in Galatians. He also mentions it throughout his other letters, and one of the most intriguing things he says about peace (in my opinion) is found in Philippians.

Rejoice in the Lord always. I will say it again: Rejoice!
Let your gentleness be evident to all.
The Lord is near. Do not be anxious about anything,
but in everything, by prayer and petition,
with thanksgiving, present your requests to God.
And the peace of God, which transcends all

understanding, will guard your hearts and
your minds in Christ Jesus.

—Philippians 4:4–7

Don't miss the end of the last verse. God's peace will guard our hearts and our minds in Christ Jesus.

The peace that comes from God is beyond our comprehension. God's peace stands sentry over our hearts and minds, protecting us from the demons of worry and anxiety.

I have experienced this peace first hand. This kind of peace comes without you trying to have it. Peace just happens.

April 2, 2010

April 2 (yesterday) was the one month anniversary of the surgery, and by all accounts I think I'm doing well. More specifically, I've made it through the healing of the incisions on the top of my head (where they drilled the holes), and now I'm in "wait and see" mode for what happens next.

For better or worse, my sense of humor seems to be normal (well, okay, it's never been normal). A couple of things I've noticed ... the short-term memory loss that I was seeing at 2 weeks seems to have dissipated. I think I'm remembering about as well as I was before (at least as far as I can remember).

The medication schedule seems more sensitive, more in flux. I can go longer between doses than I was doing beforehand, but the drop in going from "on" to "off" is a LOT quicker. If I don't time a dose right, I'm in "off" mode quicker than you can say boo.

Yeah, I'm still humming in my sleep. Last night (well this morning) I woke up humming "Christ the Lord Is Risen Today." What a great way to wake up!

One thing that is noticeably absent is my night screaming. So far, in the one month since surgery, I haven't woken up from nightmares and screaming ... that was something that was happening at least once every couple of weeks.

I recently returned from a trip with our church youth group to NYC. I was concerned that I might scream in the middle of the night, scaring the daylights out of my youth roommates. But it didn't happen, and I'm glad.

A couple of years ago, when I went to the NABBA (North American Brass Band) championships in Louisville, KY, I roomed with one of the other tuba players in our band (Triangle Brass Band), and I woke up screaming in the middle of the night. Of course it woke him up too.

Anyway ... still humming along.

I've had a few times where I still felt confused when trying to decide between options and in arranging logistics ...

I'm still more dyskinetic ... if I take a dose a bit too soon, I'm twitching more than I was before. I don't know if these things are good or bad yet ... just recording some data points. Meanwhile, the tuba still works, and our church orchestra will be rocking tomorrow morning. I can't wait!

Another Grandma

My other grandmother—my dad's mom—became blind shortly after my grandfather died in 1984. Grandma (we called her GG, since she was the great-grandmother to my kids) stayed in good spirits, though it was hard for her to adjust to losing her eyesight. Fast forward to 1995, and GG was told by doctors that her heart valves had failed and that she either needed surgery or that she would die within about 3 weeks. The surgery promised to be painful and the doctors said she had maybe a 20% chance of surviving the surgery.

She decided to not go through with the surgery. I flew out to Omaha to say good-bye to her. We spent a wonderful weekend together, with a lot of laughter and a lot of prayer. Because of her upbringing, she was accustomed to showing about as much emotion as a turnip. But when I said good-bye to her at the end of the weekend, she was crying. So was I. I flew home, and then a couple of days later she called to tell me that she decided to go forward with the surgery; she wasn't done living yet.

She had the surgery. They gave her new valves that were guaranteed for 10 years. She lived another five years beyond the guarantee of the valves, passing away in 2010 at the age of 101.

Her context was this: life is good, today is the best day she's ever had, and tomorrow is a new day.

Parkinson's has been handed to me. I could whine or I could be grateful for how it shows me that God is working in my life. Are there challenges? Certainly! Is it a great witnessing opportunity? You'd better believe it!

It's here that remembering Psalm 139 can really help.

For you created my inmost being;
you knit me together in my mother's womb.

> I praise you because I am fearfully and wonderfully
> made; your works are wonderful, I know that full well.
>
> —Psalm 139:13–14

I am humbly assured knowing that the same God who created the universe also created me.

Because of Parkinson's Disease, I stutter terribly, even when I use notes or memorize what I'm going to say. I am embarrassed and frustrated when I open my mouth to talk and no words come out. When my medication isn't working—and sometimes even when it is working—I shuffle my feet, I'm stiff, I lose my balance, and I drool. Parkinson's has other glamorous symptoms as well, including constipation, incontinence, and the possibility of hallucinations and obsessive behavior.

But I remember Psalm 139. I know that it is God, the Creator, the Supreme Ruler of the Universe, who knit me together. This same God who cares about the lilies of the field also cares about me. This same God sent his Son to die just for me.

If that doesn't give me a feeling of joy, nothing will.

Suppose you have a little Hot Wheel or Matchbox car, a red Corvette for example. As a child you spent hours at a time rolling it around on your bedroom floor, pretending it was real. That red Corvette was your favorite childhood toy. Then, one day, there's a knock on the door, and a stranger announces that you have won an actual brand new red Corvette, a real car. The only catch is that you have to give him your toy car. It's a no-brainer, right?

Yes, it's hard when we suffer in our life here on earth. Our life here, though, is but a toy when compared to the reality of eternity that we'll get to spend with the Good Shepherd.

Joy

Tucked away at the tail end of the little book of Habakkuk is this not-so-little gem, a word of encouragement for all of us. Have you ever had a bad day? Listen to this excerpt from the third chapter of Habakkuk, as presented by Eugene Peterson.

> Though the cherry trees don't blossom
> and the strawberries don't ripen,
> Though the apples are worm-eaten
> and the wheat fields stunted,
> Though the sheep pens are sheepless
> and the cattle barns empty,
> I'm singing joyful praise to God.
> I'm turning cartwheels of joy to my Savior God.
> Counting on God's rule to prevail,
> I take heart and gain strength.
> I run like a deer.
> I feel like I'm king of the mountain!
> —Habakkuk 3:17–19[1]

It sounds like a tough season to be a farmer—the crops have all failed and the livestock is gone, and yet the writer of Habakkuk is singing joyful praise and turning cartwheels of joy to God! Why? It says why in the next verse. The writer is counting on God's rule to prevail. He is depending on God. This gives him motivation and strength; this gives him swiftness; this makes him feel like royalty, knowing that the very God who created him is also taking care of him.

---

1   Peterson, Eugene H. The Message: The Bible in Contemporary Language. Colorado Springs: NavPress, 2002

Perhaps this passage is what Paul and Silas were remembering as they sang hymns of praise when they were in prison (see Acts 16:21–25).

Note that Habakkuk doesn't say anything about waiting until God makes things right first before we will all sing praise. Whether things are made right or not, we will sing praise and rejoice anyway. We know he will make things right, in his time, in his way.

Habakkuk isn't the only place in the Bible that talks about singing praise. Remember the passage from Philippians we read a few pages ago?

"Rejoice in the Lord always ... do not be anxious about anything," wrote Paul. How often is always? It's, uh, all the time. What does the "in the Lord" part have to do with anything? That's the basis for our rejoicing; that's the reason we can lift up our hands and say, "Thank you!"

Do not be anxious about anything. Being anxious is different than being eager. Eager means excited, anticipating, looking forward to something. Anxious means that you are worried about something.

What part of "Rejoice always" do I have trouble understanding? It's easy to rejoice when everything is going my way. When adversity strikes, or when I don't have my way, why do I whine or complain?

Last summer, when our church sent a group of 50 people for our annual expedition on the Appalachia Service Project, I had the privilege of working on a home for a man whom I will call Bill. Our team of seven people helped build a wheelchair ramp for Bill, an unemployed truck driver. Let me tell you a little bit about Bill.

Living in an old, small mobile home with a sturdy front porch attached, Bill had one light bulb that worked. That was in the living room. The other bulbs had electrical wiring problems that prevented them from functioning. Bill wasn't married, but he had two children of his own; and, in fact, Bill had recently become a grandfather.

Bill wasn't physically able to do much of the work that week, but he sat on the porch just about every minute that we were there, encouraging us, laughing with us, and helping where he could. Bill had, in his words, "come to Jesus" about two years earlier. When Bill wasn't helping us or talking, he was reading his Bible. He had a continual smile on his face, and his favorite topic of conversation was Jesus, specifically how Jesus had helped him turn his life around. Bill had dabbled in alcohol, drugs, and cock fighting, but that turned around when he "got religion."

When our van would show up each morning, Bill would still be inside his house, asleep. He would eventually wake up and come out on the porch in his wheelchair. He would greet us with "good morning," and usually he added, "This is a day that the Lord has made."

"You know, I ain't got much," Bill said, pointing behind himself to his home. "This here is all I have, but God is taking care of me. He is looking out for me. I am thankful for what the Lord has given me."

His remarkable faith—and the attitude it created inside him—helped him overcome the curve balls that life had thrown at him. See, Bill had some health issues.

Born with some heart irregularities, Bill has a pace maker that he has worn for years. When he was in his mid-thirties, Bill had an accident that required six vertebrae in his back to be reconstructed. Wait, that's not all. Somewhere along the way, Bill developed diabetes, and a side effect of diabetes was that a wound in his leg didn't heal properly; Bill contracted gangrene and had to have the leg amputated.

Sometimes people who have lived a long life can handle the adversity late in life. Bill was 40 years old when I met him.

Bill and I had a chance to talk a fair amount that week. He never expressed anger; he never indicated that he was depressed; he never blamed or questioned God for anything that had happened to him. Talking to him, looking into those deep eyes, Bill's life was grounded in Christ. He had a relationship with Jesus that he was clinging to, and it gave him a peace along with the ability to experience the joy of living each day. I've known people in far better shape, health-wise and economically, who cursed God for their misfortunes. If anybody deserved to be angry with God and angry with life, Bill did. But he wasn't angry with God, and he wasn't angry with life.

Bill didn't witness with fancy words or by pounding people on the head with his Bible. Bill witnessed by how he was living his life. Bill witnessed by showing that in the face of monstrous trials and difficulties in life, Jesus can provide the joy and hope that we need. When I feel like whining about Parkinson's Disease, I think about Bill and what he is going through, and I realize that I have no right to ever complain about anything.

Look at the first couple of verses from the Habakkuk passage again, this time from the New International Version.

> Though the fig tree does not bud
> and there are no grapes on the vines,
> though the olive crop fails
> and the fields produce no food,
> though there are no sheep in the pen
> and no cattle in the stalls,
> yet I will rejoice in the Lord,
> I will be joyful in God my Savior.
> —Habakkuk 3:17–18 NIV

What problems are you facing today? Are you waiting for God to fix everything before you rejoice in him? Or are you going to praise him, regardless?

When Catastrophe Strikes

My cousin Linda was beautiful, smart, witty, funny, and fun-loving. She was a go-getter, someone who knew how to get things done. When I was nine and she was thirteen, her family visited us at Christmas, and it was then that I discovered that first cousins are not allowed to marry each other. I was so disappointed.

Linda died of AIDS in 1994. Her story is a tragic one, and it breaks my heart every time I think of it. As a happy, newly married couple, Linda and her husband Michael were thriving in New York City. Shortly after their wedding, though, Linda's husband was told he had cancer of the liver. This was back in the early 1980s, before hospitals knew to test blood for HIV.

Yes, you guessed it … Linda's husband received a massive number of blood transfusions. On the day of his funeral, doctors told Linda that she had contracted HIV.

Linda put up a valiant and courageous fight, refusing to wallow in self-pity. She and another HIV-infected woman formed Women at Risk (WAR) to raise AIDS awareness, and Linda was heavily involved in speaking engagements and writing about her story until the very end.

Linda chose to live her life to the fullest, to make the best of the situation. She was a light, a candle of inspiration to all those around her. Linda even put a personal ad in the Los Angeles Times, saying that she was single with HIV and she was interested in dating. She married again, just a few months before her death.

We prayed and prayed and prayed for Linda, but she was not healed. The prayer was not answered. Why? Or perhaps the prayer was answered but the answer was "no." Again, why?

I don't know. She was so talented, so gifted. Her abilities could have been used in so many ways. Why wasn't her life spared?

No answer I give will ever provide solace for her parents. There are no magic words; there is no panacea to set things right again. It's not something I can ignore. I know that these horrible things happen; but I also know that we serve a loving Creator God. How do we reconcile those two facts?

Only a week before his arrest and crucifixion, Jesus had ridden into town on a donkey, with crowds of people lined up along the street and shouting, "Hosannah!" How could the disciples reconcile that grand entrance with the fact that Jesus was put to death only a few days later? Their dreams had been shattered, or so they thought. Their darkest hour turned out to be the foundation of the Christian church.

Tomorrow is Easter and it will be a time of celebration, joy, and praise. The very first "day before Easter" was a time of darkness, uncertainty, failure, and fear.

Who was this man, Jesus Christ, whom the disciples had been following for three years? He had performed miracles, he had given words of wisdom, and he had seemed to bring purpose to their lives. He had spoken up against the religious rulers of the day, and on the mountaintop with Peter, James, and John, this man Jesus had been in the company of Elijah and Moses.

They believed they had seen the very face of God.

They had. They just stopped believing it when their world seemingly fell apart, when their Messiah was crucified in a horrible death.

The disciples had seen enough in their three years with Jesus to know that God works in mysterious ways. But, somehow, they didn't make all the connections to the words Jesus had told them beforehand, about his needing to be killed and that he would rise three days later. It didn't fit the disciples' views of a rational world.

Life usually doesn't go quite the way we plan. Sometimes it's dramatically different.

Have you ever wanted to be able to go back in time and change things that have happened, change bad decisions you've made, change how things are? I know I have.

Regardless, remember this: God is in charge. He is in control, and he loves you more than you will ever comprehend.

You know, it takes more than a little courage to admit that you can't do it on your own. In our day and age of self sufficiency and independence, it's hard sometimes to confess that we need help. Not only do I lean on God, I am totally dependent on him. He is my Creator. He is my Savior. He is my Friend.

If I were the only sinner in the world, God would still have sent Jesus to die on the cross for me. He loves me that much.

When all is dark and dreary, when it feels as though there's no hope, when it feels as if your carriage is stuck in the mud and the strongest horses in the world can't pull you out, remember that God is there. He's got the heavy horses.

He's the one you need at the plate when it's the bottom of the ninth and you're down, 4–2.

He's the one to give the ball to when it's fourth and goal and you're down by five.

Tomorrow morning, Easter morning, will be a time to rejoice. Life is good when you let God be part of yours. Life is hard sometimes, sure. But life is good.

Courage

Wisps of steam rise from my coffee cup early on this Thursday morning. Inspired with this blank page on my screen, there's so much I want to say. I've caught glimpses of the meaning of life; I've seen shadows, figures moving in the night, apparitions from the past or the future somehow, furtively, sneaking through the backdrop of my mind; and I believe, more and more, that I'm getting an understanding of the problem of pain, the solution to suffering.

I am no theologian. I am no expert on anything, really. I am just me. I am just Joel.

However, I am compelled to write this for a couple of reasons. First, my bout with Parkinson's Disease qualifies me as being an individual who is battling some kind of chronic illness. Second, through observations from close friends and family, I have long been made aware of my unique attitude, my enthusiasm for life.

We all have choices to make. We don't have control over everything in our lives, but we choose certain things. To a great extent, we can also choose our attitudes.

Each of us has something to deal with, some nemesis that bares its fangs at us whenever it can. Perhaps an illness is threatening your retirement plans, your financial security, or maybe even your marriage. Perhaps it is the death of a loved one. Perhaps it is a job loss or a divorce. Whatever is going on in your life, you still need to get up every morning and try your best to function.

God is my reason for living. God has provided me with the perspective I need in order to continue my life. God has shown me that his promises are true, and God has provided me with the enthusiasm and motivation I need to keep going, one day at a time.

Here's the deal. I don't ascribe to the abundant living theology. That is, I don't believe for an instant that if you follow Christ with your whole heart, life will be easy and you will be blessed with gobs of money. Nowhere in the Bible does it say that, though people have twisted verses out of context.

What keeps me going? There are two things. First, I know that God is taking care of me. Second, I know that what God has awaiting us after this short life here on earth is far more wonderful, more amazing, than anything I could possibly imagine. God loves me. I am a child of God.

I am out of work. I have no job, and at this point it will be nearly impossible for me to find work that provides medical coverage. This, of course, has added tremendous stress at home.

Lord Jesus, I need you.

The thing is, I know deep in my heart that Jesus's promises are real. They're not metaphorical. Give us this day our daily bread ... I don't care at this point if it's whole wheat or rye or pumpernickel or white bread. I don't care if it's in an oblong or a round loaf, sliced or not. I know that God is going to see me through this.

When Joshua took over for Moses, just before the Hebrew nation entered the promised land after 40 years of wandering in the desert, he knew it was going to be tough. Wait—we're talking about the promised land. Wasn't that supposed to be the abundant life, the land of milk and honey? Well, yes and no. The promised land didn't come for free. Battles needed to be fought, and hardships had to be endured. Joshua needed to depend on God.

Both Joshua and the Hebrew nation needed encouragement. Before he died, Moses told the people of Israel to have courage.

> Then Moses went out and spoke these words
> to all Israel ..."Be strong and courageous.
> Do not be afraid or terrified because of them,
> for the LORD your God goes with you;
> he will never leave you nor forsake you."
>
> —Deuteronomy 31:1,6

Then, in Deuteronomy 31:7–8, Moses told Joshua to be courageous. And Joshua then heard it again, this time directly from God:

> Be strong and courageous. Do not be terrified;
> do not be discouraged, for the LORD
> your God will be with you wherever you go.
>
> —Joshua 1:9b

The Hebrew nation then told their new leader to be courageous, in Joshua 1:16–18. They also pledged their obedience to Joshua at that point. Do you think Joshua got the point? I do. In fact, later on, in Joshua 10:25–26, he ended up telling the Hebrew nation the same thing they had told him earlier.

I don't have all the answers. I'm not a smooth-talking theologian. I'm a stutterer. I'm not suave—I can't dance—and I'm not sophisticated. I don't know the latest of anything; I'm not current in my knowledge of pop culture; I don't have the latest technologies; and I'm not cool. Sometimes it's as if I don't know anything.

I know what's important though. I know God loves me. I know there are reasons that life can be painfully difficult. All I can do is lift my arms, singing praise to God. He is worthy to be worshiped. He is the one.

Do I want this disease to be removed from me? You bet I do. Will I praise God, whether I'm healed or not? You bet I will.

What about the horrible things that happen? What about children who die? What about children who are left without a mother or father? Again, I don't have the answers. All I can say is this. Life is short; life is incredibly short. When measured against all of eternity, our life here on earth is but a blip.

God has something wonderful in store for us. In John 14, Jesus says that he is preparing a room for each of us. In Revelation, we see a glimpse of what heaven is like.

If our suffering draws us closer to God, and if it breaks us so completely that we are humbled into a total lack of self-worth, then our hearts are ready for God.

Don't ever, ever, ever, ever believe for one moment that God doesn't love you. He knit you together; he knew you before you were born. He has plans for you.

> "For I know the plans I have for you," declares the LORD,
> "plans to prosper you and not to harm
> you, plans to give you hope and a future.
> Then you will call upon me and come and pray to me,
> and I will listen to you. You will seek me and find me
> when you seek me with all your heart. I will be
> found by you," declares the LORD, "and will bring
> you back from captivity. I will gather you from
> all the nations and places where I have banished you,"
> declares the LORD, "and will bring you back to the place
> from which I carried you into exile."
>
> —Jeremiah 29:11–14

Am I an expert on suffering? No way. The struggles I've gone through with Parkinson's Disease are trivial compared to so many other things out there. Even so, I think I'm qualified to ask a basic question.

If I am suffering, am I making good use of the opportunity?

Yes, it is an opportunity. It is a time for rethinking priorities. It is a time for reflection. It is a time for renewing my relationship with God. It is a time for sharing with others who are dealing with their own problems.

The deeper the pit, the stronger the urgency to find a way out. The more intense the struggle, the more heightened the awareness of the need for help. It's not until we reach rock-bottom that we fully understand we cannot do this on our own. We need a savior. We need God.

As the deer pants for streams of water,
so my soul pants for you, O God.
My soul thirsts for God, for the living God.
When can I go and meet with God?
My tears have been my food day and night,
while men say to me all day long, "Where is your God?"
Why are you downcast, O my soul?
Why so disturbed within me?
Put your hope in God, for I will yet praise him,
my Savior and my God.

—Psalm 42:1–3,5

Here is David in near despair; he's mourning, oppressed, physically and mentally suffering, and he asks his own soul, "Hey, what's up with this? Put your hope in God! Before everything is said and done, I'm going to praise him, for he is my Savior. He is my God." David is making the choice that he is going to praise God regardless.

What do you do—where do you turn—when the bottom seems to drop out of everything that you hold near and dear. Do you ask, "Why am I going through this?" Who knows except God? He's in charge. Trust him.

VI

Living in a Fallen World

Has this world been so kind to you
that you should leave with regret?
There are better things ahead
than any we leave behind.

C.S. Lewis

September 2, 2010 (6 Months)

Today is September 2, 2010, exactly six months following the surgery for CERE-120-09. How am I feeling? Well, at the moment I'm "on" and the time is 10:10 in the morning. I feel great.

Thirty minutes ago, I would have answered that I'm "off" and I feel horrid. Life is a roller coaster sometimes. Life is not perfect—after all, we live in a fallen world, don't we?

I have to be patient. I want so badly to be healed. I want this to be instant. It's not instant, though. The good things in life rarely are. As far as I can tell, there have been no changes physically, cognitively, or otherwise. I do have an exam coming up at Duke on Monday, and we'll see what they say.

When I wake up in the morning I take an assessment of where things are. I test my balance, my flexibility, and my strength. I keep waiting for that morning when my eyes pop open, I leap out of bed, and I find myself speaking like William F. Buckley, running like Jim Ryun, and writing like Ray Bradbury.

For that matter, I want to bench press like Ndamukong Suh, sing like Frank Sinatra, and play tuba like Roger Bobo.

Then I realize ... wait a minute ... I'm living in the greatest country on earth with a health care system that (so far) still meets my needs. I have the freedom to write what I want and to set my own goals.

Whether the surgery works or not (and I really hope it does), I have nothing to complain about.

I have a family that loves me, siblings who love me, and countless friends who love me and are pulling and praying for me.

Some days are a lot tougher than other days, but every day is a good day. This is a day that the Lord has made. I will rejoice and be glad in it.

My nephew told my sister the other day, rather matter-of-factly, that "Uncle Joel will be healed six months after the surgery."

I wanted to wake up this morning with a feeling that I should be dancing. I wanted to be like Gene Wilder in "Charlie and the Chocolate Factory," doing somersaults and singing. I wanted to wake up singing songs from "Oklahoma!" or "The Sound of Music."

Instead, I woke up feeling like the guy in the old Spike Jones song, "I haven't been home for three whole nights—last night, tonight, and tomorrow."

Oh, don't get me wrong. When I wake up, I'm happy. But when I wake up, my body doesn't want to move. After lying in bed all night, my body is stiff. It aches as I sit up and put my feet on the floor. The first stepping upward to a standing position hurts—literally, it hurts—and I find myself hoping that I don't fall down backwards into bed and have to try it again.

The first few steps toward the bathroom door are slow. I mentally tell my legs to move, and then my feet shuffle, leaving a trail in the carpet that looks like cross country ski tracks in the snow. As my body leans forward, my feet go faster and faster with the shuffle, trying to keep up with the rest of the body so that I don't topple over. Once I get started, the tough part is then stopping.

The toilet is just to the left of the far wall in the bathroom. The far wall also has a large window. One of my goals in life is to not go through that window.

It takes 30 to 40 minutes on average for the morning medication to kick in. This morning I took the parcopa first, and then I ate a bowl of cereal for breakfast before taking the rest of the medications. That was a mistake. I ended up being "off" for an additional two hours or so this morning.

So I find myself trying to spread the medicines out a bit, with the hope that eventually I'll be able to drop them entirely. For three nights in a row earlier this week, I dropped my evening parcopa. However, last night it all seemed to catch up with me. I finally needed a parcopa to make it through the evening.

I did go to a Bible study at church last night, and I stayed awake for the whole thing. I'm doing well with staying awake this week. I know that sounds like a minor, trivial thing. I tell you, though, it's so unusual for me to stay awake in ANY meeting.

Yesterday morning, I ran for 1.5 miles with my younger daughter; then, last night, I ran for 2.5 miles with my oldest son. It's feeling good to get more exercise than I've gotten in a while.

My body will toggle between "off" and "on" today, though it should be mostly "on." I wish it were all the way "on."

So, with all of this, I'm convinced that a sense of humor is needed to be able to roll with the punches. Can you imagine if this mortal life here on earth were all there was? Still, even knowing that our earthly existence is relatively short, the prayer that Paul gives to the people of Ephesus can encourage us.

For this reason I kneel before the Father, from whom his whole family in heaven and on earth derives its name.

I pray that out of his glorious riches he may strengthen you with power through his Spirit in your inner being, so that Christ may dwell in your hearts through faith.

And I pray that you, being rooted and established in love, may have power, together with all the saints, to grasp how wide and long and high and deep is the love of Christ, and to know this love that surpasses knowledge—that you may be filled to the measure of all the fullness of God.

Now to him who is able to do immeasurably more than all we ask or imagine, according to his power that is at work within us, to him be glory in the church and in Christ Jesus throughout all generations, for ever and ever! Amen.

—Ephesians 3:14–21

One Happy Dog

In a perfect world, we would make the right decisions. We wouldn't rush; we would think things through; and we would do the right thing every time. This isn't a perfect world.

The date was January 1st. The year was 1974. I was partially awake, mostly relaxed, completely horizontal, and full from the roasted turkey we had devoured only two hours earlier. I was watching one of the bowl games on television. Max was out in his backyard pen.

Half dachshund and half basset hound, Max weighed in at 29 pounds. He had a stocky chest, strong legs, and a thin waist, and we worked hard at not overfeeding him. He mostly ate dry dog food, but on holidays and on his birthday we would give him table left-overs as a treat.

"Joel, could you take the turkey scraps out to Max during the next commercial?" Dad asked. I waited until a commercial and then dashed into the kitchen.

There, on the table, I spied the big roasting pan with pieces of turkey. I grabbed the pan, leaned it onto my hip so that I could open the back door—the pan was heavy and I reasoned that the turkey carcass was probably also in the pan—and I stepped outside.

I carried the pan across the backyard to Max's pen, walking quickly because I wanted to get back before the game resumed. As I approached the pen, I heard the eager and energetic pitter-patter of Max's footsteps on the concrete slab and I knew the smell of the turkey was exciting him.

I reached over the fence and poured the contents of the roasting pan into Max's food bowl. The carcass and scraps were piled up so high that it wouldn't all fit into Max's modest sized bowl. It was getting dark, but still I could see Max's tail wagging so fast that if he were a helicopter he would have lifted straight up in the air.

I had never seen Max that thrilled.

I ran back inside, set the pan on the counter, and found my still warm spot on the couch as I continued watching the game.

A couple of hours later, Dad went into the kitchen to make a sandwich for dinner. His voice rang out, "Where's the turkey?"

I responded, "What turkey?"

He replied, "The turkey that was in the roasting pan."

My heart sank faster than an anvil in a swimming pool. I gasped, "Uh oh," and in one motion I grabbed a flashlight, opened the back door, and leaped out into the cool night.

"Max! Max!" I cried out. Again I heard his footsteps, only this time they weren't prancing. He was moving more slowly than a young couple at a high school prom dancing to the first half of Freebird. I directed the beam of light to his empty food bowl, which was completely licked clean. Then I focused the light on Max. He was huge. His normally lean waist was as wide as his chest, and he had the biggest smile on his face that I've ever seen.

I walked slowly back inside. Dad was still standing there, holding two slices of bread and hoping that what he was guessing had happened hadn't really happened.

But it had.

Next to Dad, on the counter, was a small cereal bowl with the table scraps of turkey, perhaps a quarter pound of meat at the most. That's what Dad had wanted me to give to Max.

I wish I could say that I was following my routine and that someone had always cut away all the turkey meat from the carcass right after dinner, but that is not true. I just wasn't thinking. I was in a hurry, and even though I noticed the roasting pan was heavy, I didn't stop to ask.

The family had to improvise for dinner that night and for lunch the next day. Max, meanwhile, got approximately fifteen pounds of that twenty-two pound bird. He didn't touch food again for a couple of days.

In a fallen world, things go haywire. Simple tasks become complex; complex tasks blow up. Sometimes the results are comical and relatively harmless; sometimes they're not. We can be careful, but there's a reason that Murphy's Law ("If something can go wrong, it will") exists. On this side of heaven, it's the norm.

The Day I Fell into the Pond

Have you ever had one of those days where you feel so good that you find yourself wondering how long it's going to last? Glorious days that seem to come to life from a Norman Rockwell painting, postcard days that could have been in the background when the cowboy Curly in "Oklahoma!" was singing "Oh What a Beautiful Morning," days that might someday be featured in ESPN's Top Ten Days Ever—days like that are rare, few and far between.

Shortly after moving down here to North Carolina, I was having one of those kind of days. At least, the first half of the day had been glorious, and all I had to do was to hang on for the remaining few hours and it would be one of the best days in my then still young life.

The sky was blue, I loved my job (working for Data General, the company featured in Tracy Kidder's Pulitzer Prize winning book, *Soul of a New Machine*), and I was still feeling the newlywed glow—it was just a day where I felt great. I hadn't won the lottery or anything like that, but I could walk into my office and yell, "Wheeeee," because I was having so much fun.

You would be hard pressed to find a better thing to do on a day like that than go with your colleagues on a picnic lunch to the breathtakingly beautiful Duke Gardens! The azaleas were in full bloom, the bluebirds were whistling on my shoulder, and Mary Poppins was singing that *supercalifragilesticexpyalidocious* song (hmm, my spell checker doesn't like that word). All was right with the world.

After lunch, my manager Scott suggested we extend the lunch hour and throw the Frisbee on the large open field in the gardens. I had brought my Frisbee just in case, so I was ready for some fun. Scott, Ben, and I were playing, making beautiful long throws that were highlighted by the sunshine glinting off the Frisbee as it whirled against the deep blue Carolina sky. Off in the distance, a man on a tractor was mowing the lawn. The fresh smell of cut grass filled the air.

I threw to Scott, Scott threw to Ben, and Ben threw to me; and then again, I threw to Scott, Scott threw to Ben, and Ben threw ... way over my head.

I was in pretty good shape in those days, so I turned and ran, determined to show off my speed and athletic prowess by chasing down the spinning disk. I saw it ahead of me, moving quickly but staying aloft, and I knew with confidence I'd be able to track it. I kept my focus on it in case it wanted to start drifting to the left or right.

The Frisbee and I were converging. I lengthened my stride a bit to make sure I would get there, and the Frisbee slowly began lowering from the sky. I ran and ran and—

Whoa!

There, immediately in front of me, was the big goldfish pond. I was still running full speed and this pond was not more than five feet from me. I slammed on the brakes and stopped right on the very edge of the pond.

Here came the Frisbee. I reached up, stretching my arms, legs, and torso as far as I could, and I whisked the Frisbee out of the air.

Uh oh.

I had stretched perhaps a bit too far. I was leaning forward just an iota, just a smidgen, but just enough that I knew I was headed for some water.

In that fraction of a second before I hit water, I analyzed the situation. I couldn't see the bottom of the murky goldfish pond, but I guessed that it couldn't be more than two feet deep. Not bad, I reasoned. My feet and legs prepared for the landing, anticipating ending up about two feet below the water surface.

I was wrong.

The pond was approximately four feet deep. I ended up tumbling all the way under water, completely submerged. What a shock!

I quickly climbed back out of the pond. Yes, I had caught the frisbee and was still hanging on to it.

Scott was doubled over in laughter. Ben was doubled over in laughter. And the man who had been on the riding lawn mower was off the machine, on the ground, laughing so hard that he was pounding the grass with his fist.

It was one of those moments when you try to laugh at yourself because everyone else is already laughing at you, but the self-laugh comes out as a sort of stilted, "Ha (pause) ha (pause) ha."

I spent the rest of the afternoon totally soaked and dripping in my office. Fortunately I had no meetings that afternoon. I don't think I got much work done ... I was pondering about how the day had been beautifully perfect up to that point. And I wondered ...

In "Oklahoma!," right after he sings the song about the beautiful morning, does he ride into a low-hanging branch and get knocked off his horse?

Or in "The Sound of Music," as Julie Andrews is running across the mountain meadow, does she trip and tumble down a steep slope (presumably colliding with the nun who is climbing every mountain)?

I usually have an optimistic outlook on life, and I tend to enjoy most every moment. But when things are going too well, I start hedging my bets and looking around for that pond. If it's around somewhere, I'm sure to fall in.

Soapy Tales

I n an imperfect world, even the best of intentions can lead to disastrous results ... especially when we take a guess and it's the wrong choice.

Before I went to college, I learned how to wash and iron my own laundry. I was so good at it that for a while in college I even ironed my tee-shirts. I remember Mom telling me to always be sure that I used laundry detergent and to never ever use dish soap in the laundry. She didn't really tell me why.

I landed my first job out of school with GE in Schenectady, New York. It was a great job in a great town, and I thoroughly enjoyed the three years I spent there. During my last two years in Schenectady, I rented a house and had a roommate named Jeff.

One Saturday, Jeff had to go in to work, and I played the part of the domesticated roommate. I tidied the living room, took out the garbage, washed some dishes, and loaded up the dishwasher with the plates that were in the sink.

I was dismayed to find that the dishwasher detergent box was empty, and then I remembered I had used it up last time but had forgotten to buy more. I figured on a Saturday morning the grocery stores would be packed, and I was thinking it would be at least a 45–minute proposition to go to the store and back. I really wanted to get back to the book I had been reading, so I looked around to see if I could find other soap to use.

Ah! There on the shelf was a bottle of dish soap. Then I heard Mom's voice in the back of my head, "Don't ever use dish soap for doing laundry."

But hey, I wasn't doing laundry. I was going to run the dishwasher. If you couldn't use dish soap in the dishwasher, well, that just didn't sound right.

I filled up the little dispenser thing in the dishwasher door, closed it, and turned it on.

Happy that the house was clean, I went back to the living room and continued reading.

It was perhaps ten minutes later that I heard a sound somewhat similar to the familiar Snap, Crackle, and Pop of the old Rice Krispies commercials. I put my book down a moment and listened, and then I heard the dishwasher do its gurgle thing. Oh, I must have just been hearing water coming into or out of the machine, I reasoned. I continued reading.

Another few minutes later, I heard the sound again. It was louder. I was sitting with my back to the kitchen. The doorway to the kitchen had no door; it was an open entrance.

I turned around to see what might be happening. What I saw was a glacier-like layer of soap suds, maybe eight inches thick, oozing from the kitchen, through the doorway, and into the living room. Oh no!

I leaped off the couch and ran to the kitchen doorway. The entire kitchen floor was covered.

Taking my shoes off, I quickly waded through the soap sud glacier to the dishwasher, turned it off, and pondered my next step. I ran down into the basement, found a bucket and the mop, and ran back up to the kitchen.

I filled up several buckets of soap suds and dumped them down the sink, but then the sink filled up with soap and it wouldn't go down the drain. I ran water into the sink, but that only seemed to create more bubbles! So I took buckets of soap suds and poured them down the toilet, and then more buckets were poured into the bathtub, and finally I poured more buckets in the shower.

Remember the Lucille Ball episode when she is overwhelmed with a conveyor belt of chocolates and she ends up stuffing chocolate in her pockets, her hat, her shirt, her mouth, and anywhere else she can find? I knew exactly how Lucy felt!

There were soap suds everywhere, and for a while I thought I would never be able to get rid of them. What's more, I was embarrassed about the situation, and I wanted to get it all cleaned up before Jeff got home.

Part of the problem with trying to do this quickly though was that the plumbing just couldn't handle the volume of soap suds. Bubbles stopped going down the drain. I ended up dumping a bunch of soap bubbles behind the bushes in the backyard.

For the next thirty minutes I was pouring soap suds down any drain I could find, and I was running water and flushing toilets trying to get this spectacular mountain of soap dissolved and out of the house.

It got a little more complicated though because by the time I had gotten all the soap off the floor, there were streaks all over from the dirt that loosened up during my soap sud battle. I ended up having to scrub the kitchen floor so that it would look uniform in dirtiness (or cleanliness, rather).

I also had to scrub the toilets, the shower, and the bathtub. I never thought I was going to get done.

Just as I finished the last of the cleaning, Jeff's car pulled into the driveway, and as the back door opened I was sitting on the couch, acting deeply engrossed in the book.

The first thing he said when he stepped into the kitchen was, "Wow!"

I asked, "What?"

Jeff said, "Thanks for scrubbing the kitchen floor! I had been thinking about doing that. It looks great!"

All I could manage was, "Thanks Jeff."

He went upstairs, and a moment later I heard another, "Oh man!"

"What?" I asked again.

"You cleaned the toilet. And the bathtub. And the shower!"

"Well, yeah, I ... uh ... I kind of had to," I humbly replied. I told him the whole story, and he laughed and then I laughed. I don't know why I had been embarrassed about the episode, except that, well, I probably should have known better.

A few months ago, my fourteen-year-old daughter and I were cleaning the kitchen.

"Dad?"

"Yes, Laura?"

"We're out of dishwasher soap. Can we just use dish soap?"

I smiled and said, "I've got a story for you."

It does seem to me that not being able to use dish soap in a dishwasher is someone's idea of trying to make this world more complicated than it needs to be. Life is like that. I discovered late one night that even though my tube of toothpaste looks nearly identical to my tube of cream for athlete's foot, they don't taste the same. I also found out one Saturday morning that the jar of homemade maple syrup in the refrigerator was the same size and color as the jar of homemade clove mouthwash that my oldest daughter had made. Now I know why clove-flavored pancake syrup is not a hot-selling item at the grocery store.

Heaven

Why would the God who created you, the same God who knows the number of hairs on your heads, throw you to the wolves and let you hang out to dry?

Does he really do that? I am not even going to attempt to answer that question here. I am no theologian, and this is a question that has troubled the best minds for centuries. There are some who believe that God is totally hands-off and that he sits back and allows life on earth to run its course, whatever that means. There are others who (like Job's friends) blame a man's sorrows on his own sinful behavior, while another camp says that a man's sins may be punished down through several layers of his descendants.

Anyway, all that aside, there is something even more important to mention at this point. Never, ever forget the fact that there's more to life than the tiny iota of life that we experience here on earth. No matter how bad life is—and it can be pretty rough—there's an eternity awaiting us when we leave this place.

> I consider that our present sufferings are not worth comparing with the glory that will be revealed in us.
>
> —Romans 8:18

Yes, we want to rationalize everything and try to understand God and account for all the actions of everybody, deity or human alike. The fact is, though, that our time here is brief. Time with him will be glorious. It seems the focus for most of life is on how to become successful here, the rules for living here, and all that. This is just the introduction to life. This is the primer, the "here's how I made you, here's what I expect, and let me show you how much I love you" course. Our real mission, long-term, is to praise and worship him, our Creator, Redeemer, and Comforter.

Then I saw a new heaven and a new earth, for the first heaven and the first earth had passed away,
and there was no longer any sea. I saw the Holy City, the new Jerusalem, coming down out of heaven from God, prepared as a bride beautifully dressed for her husband. And I heard a loud voice from the throne saying, 'Now the dwelling of God is with men, and he will live with them. They will be his people, and God himself will be with them and be their God. He will wipe every tear from their eyes. There will be no more death or mourning or crying or pain, for the old order of things has passed away.

—Revelation 21:1–4

I can't picture anything more glorious than being on my knees among a throng of people, praising God.

Have you ever been in a crisis, and you prayed fervently, and somehow the crisis resolved so that you were safe, your kids were safe, and your spouse was safe? What did you do then? You got down on your knees and your heart was filled with love and gratitude and praise for the Lord, and it felt so good to praise him and thank him for what he did that you thought you could stay on your knees all day doing that.

That, I think, is at least part of what heaven will be like. When we get there, we'll more fully understand the magnitude of what he has done for us. We will be so blown away that it won't occur to us that we can do anything but be on our knees offering our worship and praise to him. It's going to be amazing.

"When we've been there ten thousand years,
bright shining as the sun,
we've no less days to sing God's praise
than when we'd first begun."

(from "Amazing Grace," by John Newton)

Waiting for Christmas

We take down our Christmas tree later and later every year, and this year we had the tree up until the last day of February. We even turned it into a Valentine tree on February 14th, when my son Aaron decorated it with dozens of hearts cut from construction paper. My youngest daughter, Laura, was mortified when I mentioned the prospect of keeping the tree up until Thanksgiving.

Why keep the tree standing? Part of the deal is procrastination, gathering up enough momentum to overcome inertia and to bring down the six boxes from storage so that we can put away all the ornaments until next Christmas. Part of it, though, honestly is that we enjoy the Christmas season so much that we don't want it to end.

I love Christmas. I love the music: singing Christmas carols as a family while we set up and decorate the tree; playing the inspiring and joyful hymns in the church orchestra on Christmas Eve; and singing *Silent Night* with the rest of the congregation as we hold our candles high in the air. I love the festivities: the parties, with cookies and laughter and games; the gathering of relatives as we enjoy a big Christmas meal; the opening of presents on Christmas morning, and watching *It's a Wonderful Life* on TV. Most of all, I love the worship: reading the passage from Luke; experiencing the fellowship of friends at church; and welcoming the Christ child into our lives. Christmas is a special time as we wait expectantly for God to do his thing.

Every day should be a day of joyful expectation, shouldn't it? Maybe today is the day that Aunt Mary will bring over a strawberry pie; maybe today is the day that I'll get an email from a long lost friend; maybe today is the day that I'll be healed from Parkinson's Disease.

Most important of all, today is another opportunity for me to welcome the Christ child into my life, embracing him and allowing him to work through me.

Clearing the tree of its ornaments and putting them back in their little boxes and bags, and then into the larger boxes, is a time of celebration. We play Christmas music, we sing songs, we reminisce about the holiday that has just finished, and we enjoy the time together.

This year, as we threw the tree out into the woods to provide shelter for birds — hey, come over and I'll show you trees from the past four or five years — I realized that there were only 299 shopping days until next Christmas! Forget about this past Christmas, it's time to start preparing for the next.

As I swept up the little needles that had fallen from the tree, I was softly singing "Hark the Herald" to myself, not thinking that anyone was listening. I sang the first half of the first verse and then stopped when one of the kids came in to ask me a question. I forgot I had been singing and didn't finish the song.

A moment or two later, Laura, who was in the kitchen washing dishes, started singing right where I had left off. I joined back in, though I sang quietly so I could still hear Laura's beautiful voice.

I had many special moments during this Christmas season, times when I was overwhelmed with gratitude for all that God has done in my life. This particular moment, finishing up a verse of the song together, was one of the sweetest.

From father to child, the love of Christmas — more specifically, the worship of Jesus Christ — continues.

Glory to the newborn King!

Free Will and a Fallen World

The famous question is this: Why do bad things happen to good people. I have an answer that, to some people, may seem flippant. The answer is this: Bad things happen to good people because they do. We live in a fallen world.

C.S. Lewis once said, "The real problem is not why some pious, humble, believing people suffer, but why some do not."

That's little consolation for the child who loses his father or mother to cancer or an automobile accident, nor does it provide solace for the parent who loses a child to disease. I understand how people can lose hope in situations like that, or how people turn to any of several escapes that our society provides (and even encourages) ... sex, alcohol, drugs, etc.

However, I firmly believe that what awaits us in heaven is amazing compared to what we see here; eternal life with Jesus will be so unspeakably glorious that it will make all of our hardships here seem trivial.

Not that they are trivial. I'm not saying that. We just cannot imagine what paradise will be like, really. We do know that there will be no more tears, no more sadness.

The whole discussion of a free universe is one that has been debated for a long time. Does God cause everything to happen; does God allow everything to happen; or is God unable to control everything that happens?

You're sitting in the park with your date, a woman named Marionette, after a nice dinner and a movie. "How did you like the dinner?" you ask.

Marionette sits there in silence. Finally, you pick up the board with the strings, you move her head so she looks at you, and you say in your best ventriloquist voice, "It was wonderful, Darling."

"How about the movie? Did you like that too?" you ask.

She stays still for a few seconds longer, giving the appearance of thinking something profound. Then she turns her head again and whispers, "It was divine."

"So tell me, Marionette, about your date. Was the guy handsome, charming, and funny?"

"Don't put words in my mouth," mutters Marionette.

What you really want is for your date to like you and eventually perhaps to love you. Wouldn't it be awful if Marionette really were a marionette, incapable of her own thoughts and dreams? You could get her to say anything you wanted her to say, but it would be meaningless.

God, too, wants us to love him, but in his wisdom he gave us the complete, free choice of where our love and our allegiances lie.

A God who ruled the universe's events with dictatorial authority would be like the parent who watched his child too closely and didn't allow him to encounter adversity. The child would learn nothing and wouldn't grow emotionally or spiritually because there would be no need for it.

My wife keeps a vegetable garden during the spring, summer, and fall in North Carolina. During the winter she begins growing the plants indoors under lights to give them an early start. This protects the plants from the winter cold, snow, and ice (what little of it we do get here in the South). When spring approaches, she sets trays of the little seedlings out on the front porch during the day—for an hour or two at first, and then eventually for whole days. The plants are still protected, but they harden because of exposure to the elements. Eventually they are put out in the garden, ready to take on the cool spring nights and, later, the intense summer heat.

Don't we all want God to treat us that way in some respect? We would love to get hardened under the watchful eye of a God who is preparing us for the summer of life. Of course, we don't want to be set out during the winter before we're ready, but we also don't want to be an indoor plant the whole time—it would be difficult to grow to our full potential without the bright, shining radiance of the sun.

By now you're asking, "Well, what's the point?" The point is that adversity, tough situations, illness, disasters, and simply being in the wrong place at the wrong time can be horrific, but still God allows these things to happen. Why? I don't have the foggiest idea. I do know that somehow it all fits together in God's plan. I also know that God loves us; God wants us to grow in our love for him; and God wants us to develop to our fullest potential to serve him.

Things happen that don't make sense from our myopic perspectives. We need to trust in God's wisdom; we need to believe that he knows what's going to happen and that he allows things to happen; and we need to keep our eyes focused on the goal. Life here on earth is short; life in heaven, with him, is going to be glorious.

The other thing to consider is that maybe, just maybe, we're looking at this whole thing backward. Maybe it's not all about us. Maybe it's all about God.

The designer of the universe is not a God of whim and carelessness. Remember, God loves you unconditionally. Not only does he love you, he died for you.

> And we know that in all things God works for the good of those who love him, who have been called according to his purpose.
>
> —Romans 8:28

VII

Patience and Perseverance

But in the mud and scum of things,
There alway, alway something sings.

Ralph Waldo Emerson

So comes snow after fire, and even dragons
have their endings.

J.R.R. Tolkien

November 2, 2010

Eight months after the surgery, I still see no positive effect. Oh, every once in a while someone will comment—*Looking good today, Schnoor*—but in general I feel worse than I did back in March. My "off" times are longer, they come more quickly, I can't revert from "off" back to "on" quite as easily as I could before, and all the other symptoms are progressively going downhill.

I have a shuffle that looks like Tim Conway's old man walk; I still fall asleep in long meetings, concerts, movies, television shows, occasionally in church, or at any event where the lights are dimmed; my balance is more precarious than before; and, unfortunately, the organizational and problem-solving part of my brain seems to be getting more confused over time.

Last Friday I tried changing out the brake light bulbs in the back of my car. Both the middle "high mount" bulb and the left rear brake light were not working. The middle bulb was easy to fix, but the left rear bulb involved determining which light was the brake light and which was the tail light. I ended up replacing the turn signal light inadvertently, but I was convinced it was the brake light and I was baffled why the brake light still wasn't working.

I turn 50 in May of 2011. I used to think I would live well into my 90's. After all, my paternal grandmother lived to be 101 (and her older sister also passed away at 101). Many mornings when I wake up, though, it's a struggle to get out of bed. My body doesn't want to move.

Stuttering hasn't changed. I go to a couple of Bible studies at church during the week, and often it's embarrassing trying to say anything. My mouth will open to say a word, and nothing will come out. I sit there with my mouth open, trying to get a word out but also hoping at the same time that I don't drool.

I've read recently that in the first CERE-120 clinical trial, where two drops of the gene therapy drug were inserted, the patients are now *(after 18—24 months) finally starting to see some tangible benefits. I'm hoping and praying that this second CERE-120 clinical trial is at least as successful.*

What are some of the more intangible things to fight? Confidence is huge. I feel as though I'm in a large room, sitting on the floor with my talents and abilities surrounding me. One by one, these talents and abilities are taken away.

I used to be a good speaker. Now I stammer.

I used to be a decent tennis player—not great, but I could play pretty well. Now I struggle to keep my balance and to chase down the ball.

What I am seeing, though, is that the typical, progressive downhill descent continues. I drop from being "on" to being "off" much more quickly now; the "off" periods last longer; and the "off" periods are deeper and tougher to recover from than they earlier were.

I'm continuing to see a decline in the "executive functions" part of the brain. The past few years, it has been a challenge for me to pull together data, to keep to commitments and schedules, and to be able to focus on anything. Oh, I'm getting some tasks done, but not at the rate to which I had become accustomed.

I won't lose heart (nor should you). Compared to the first CERE-120 clinical trial, my surgery comprised more injections of the virus and in a deeper part of the brain (the substantia nigra, where the problem resides). I guess it takes a significant amount of time to repair and restore the dead or damaged dopamine-producing neurons.

The second and more important reason that I won't lose heart is because I know that God is in charge; God is in control. He is sovereign and he knows what he's doing.

This same God who created me—this same God who knew all my days even before I was born—knows what is best for me. God loves me, and if in his wisdom he says that I need to have Parkinson's Disease, who am I to argue with him?

He's right. He's always right.

Do I want to be healed? Of course!

Will it happen? I don't have a clue.

Will I praise God either way?

Yes I will. Healed or not healed, I will praise God, my Lord and Savior.

Of Fishing

Fishing has played a fairly significant role in my life in my forty some years on this planet; I've gone on numerous fishing trips; I've fished in fresh and salt water; I've had days with a bucket full of fish; I've had days with no fish; I've had days with nice sized fish; and I've had days with fish that were smaller than the lure with which they were caught. I've had one fish, two fish, and red fish. I have yet to catch a blue fish (though we do have them out here on the Carolina coast).

So it was, when my own kids became old enough to do something resembling fishing, I took them out, one by one, and taught them how to fish. I'll have to say that not all of them enjoy fishing, but they all know how to fish.

All these years, the more I thought about it, the more I realized that my dad took me fishing partly to teach me the sport, but primarily to teach me patience. There's nothing like sitting there as a four year old, waiting for that bobber to go under.

"Dad, when will a fish come?"

"You asked me that about thirty seconds ago."

"Dad, when can we go home?"

"We got here two minutes ago."

"Dad?"

"What son?"

"Your bobber went underwater. Should you reel it in?"

My dad is many things, and one of his hallmarks is patience. I know few people as patient as my father, and I had always attributed that to the fact that his father used to take him fishing, thus teaching my dad patience.

This story involves Nathan, who had just turned four.

Our house backed up to a thirty acre neighborhood lake. This was perfect for fishing from shore or for taking out the canoe. My wife and I had bought a sixteen foot fiberglass canoe shortly after we were married, and I loved (and still love) taking that thing out on the water.

One particular weekday morning, Nathan and I were both up early. I had just finished my morning reading and my cup of coffee, and Nathan asked me if we could go fishing sometime. "Why not now?" I thought to myself. I had another hour before I needed to drive to work, so I figured we could get the canoe out and fish for a little bit.

Within minutes we were out in the canoe. I rigged up my son's line with a worm and a bobber, while I was using a plastic lure on my line. I caught a small bass, and then another, all within the first ten minutes. Nathan had gotten no bites.

That's okay, I thought to myself. This will teach him patience.

As if reading my mind, he then stated, "I think I should use what you're using, Dad."

"Well Son, you don't really know how to cast yet."

"Can you teach me?"

I couldn't turn down that request. We reeled in his line; I put on a swivel and a Rapala lure with two treble hooks; and I showed him how to cast.

His first cast was actually fine. It went perhaps ten feet. He reeled in and tried again. He put a lot of effort into the second cast.

He was sitting in the front of the canoe, facing away from me, so I didn't immediately notice what had happened. I did realize though that I hadn't heard the soft splash of the lure in the water. Then I heard a little voice. "Uh oh. I'm stuck."

He turned halfway around. There, stuck in his soft sweatpants, was the lure. One treble hook was stuck in his right pant leg; the other treble hook was stuck in his left pant leg. His legs effectively were stuck together.

"Hold still, son," I commanded. "I'll come help you."

Now, I do know better than to try to move while in a canoe, but we didn't have a lot of time left, and I wanted to get this lure freed so that he could fish a little more. I lowered my center of mass and basically crawled along the bottom of the canoe until I could reach his legs.

I reached my right arm over his seat, trying to find the lure. I quickly found that my shirt sleeve had snagged on one of the treble hooks. So there I was, face down in the canoe with one arm stuck to my son's legs, which were fastened together with the lure. I was frustrated and I could feel myself getting ready to snap.

This felt like a scene with Lucille Ball or perhaps Tim Conway.

When I realized how comical it must have looked, I began laughing, and soon both my son and I were laughing as we worked to get the hooks out. Eventually, we succeeded.

At that moment, I had an epiphany.

My dad was patient, yes. But his patience wasn't because his father had taken him fishing. My dad was patient because he had taken me fishing, time and time again over all those years.

All those snagged hooks, the tangled lines, the frequent requests to change lures, and all the "I'm hungry" or "I'm thirsty" or "I'm tired" or "I have to go to the bathroom" interruptions ... all of this played together to develop a solid, rock-like patience.

Yes, my dad and I had great times together fishing, and the happy memories are countless, but God used those opportunities to bless Dad with a patience that would serve him well later in life and would be an inspiration to others. Now it was my turn to do the same thing.

We didn't catch any more fish that morning, but our fishing adventures together had started, and I looked forward to more adventures. I also looked forward to more opportunities to strengthen my own patience.

Patience

Why is waiting so hard? We are groomed for instant gratification. Our society has taught us that we should be able to have it our way. We want what we want, and we want it now. Our culture has turned us all into "our way is the only way" people. We aren't willing to wait; we aren't willing to serve; and we aren't willing to get out of our comfort zones. We have become a society of extraordinarily impatient people.

Each of us probably thinks he is immune to this pattern of thinking. Where does your impatience appear, though? Do you have an illness that has caused you to pray for healing for months or years, and you're getting tired of waiting? Do you want people at your side, serving you and catering to your every whim, but you're not getting the sympathy you think you deserve?

"That has nothing to do with being patient," you say.

But it does. Being patient means not only waiting on someone else's timetable, but waiting on someone else's to-do list, a list that perhaps looks considerably different than your own. Your set of priorities might not match the priorities of anyone else in your world.

"But isn't it really God who requires my patience," you wonder, "and not my spouse or next-door neighbor or family relative?"

Even in illness, you are accountable for your attitude and your behavior to those around you.

Why do I say that? Look at what Paul says in Romans.

Be joyful in hope; patient in affliction; faithful in prayer.

—Romans 12:12

Paul calls us to be patient in spite of whatever is troubling us, not because it is easy, but because it is the right thing to do. Like it or not, people will look to see how you respond to adversity. If you respond with bitterness, anger, impatience, or even whining and complaining, you are squelching the peace and joy that God provides.

You've been praying for healing for a long time, and it hasn't happened yet. It's all too easy to get frustrated with God and to take that out on the people around you. Impatience can lead to a short fuse, which in turn can lead to anger, arguments, and hurt feelings.

Do you remember the Hebrew nation that Moses led out of Egypt, and they wandered in the desert and ate manna for 40 years before finally making it to the promised land?

> They traveled from Mount Hor along the route
> to the Red Sea, to go around Edom.
> But the people grew impatient on the way;
> they spoke against God and against Moses,
> and said, "Why have you brought us up
> out of Egypt to die in the desert? There is no bread!
> There is no water!
> And we detest this miserable food!"
>
> —Numbers 21:4–6

They had forgotten God's promises! They had failed to remember how God had delivered them from the hands of the enemy. The parting of the Red Sea was long gone from their minds.

God is perfect; God is loving; God is just; and God is wise. Why then wouldn't he answer our prayers, which we think we deserve? Are we patient when we know that God has the ability to fix everything and yet he doesn't heal us? He is God. Trust him. He knows what he's doing.

I wake up on some days thinking, "This is it … the brain surgery is starting to kick in" (I do wonder, of course, whether "kick in" is a valid verbal phrase or if I'm really ending a sentence with a preposition). Then, on subsequent days, I'll realize that not only has the brain surgery not kicked in yet, but I'm still going downhill on this slippery slope of Parkinson's Disease.

Like the little girl in the Longfellow poem, when I'm "on" I feel very, very "on," but when I'm "off," I'm horrid.

Anyway, I am still waiting in anticipation of this CERE-120 trial really taking hold. There is promise. I am a child waiting for Christmas to come. It will come.

How different, though, are the two statements: "There is promise" and "There is a promise."

The former implies hope, a desire, a wish. The latter implies a certainty, a guarantee.

God has given us a promise of eternal life, a promise that our life here doesn't really end but that it goes on with him. I cling to that promise. That promise supersedes the promises of anything that happens here on planet earth.

Would it be nice to be healed? Yes, it would. It would be awesome. But, in the grand scheme of things, it won't hold a candle to the promise of what God has in store for us.

Learning English by the Buckets

She was old when she taught my mom English some twenty-five years earlier, so I guess that made her older than old when I sat down at my desk in her eighth grade English class in Blencoe, Iowa. The tired wood floors, the musty lockers, and the smell of fresh #2 pencil shavings set the stage for this paragon of academia.

Mrs. Akin was a tough instructor who knew how to take a class by the reins and lead it through the acrid marshes of Edgar Allen Poe, the adventurous river tales of Mark Twain, and the Martian wastelands of Ray Bradbury.

She did it all—we read the masters, we took painful stabs at creative writing, and we learned how to diagram sentences until I was convinced that I could diagram my own grandmother.

I said she was tough—she was as tough as the backside of an old goat—but she wasn't mean. She had a streak of playfulness that kept the class guessing. Still, there was no testing her authority, not if you wanted to live to see the next sunrise.

Mrs. Akin, without fail, always gave us ten or fifteen minutes at the end of class to read. She would use the opportunity to leave the room and go to the ladies room to smoke a cigar. If it was supposed to be a secret, it wasn't a well kept one. I suspected at the time that she allowed the secret to leak because it added to the mystique of her professorial persona.

Anyway, one warm spring day as we were reading a short story by James Thurber, Mrs. Akin decided the room was too warm. The old building had no air conditioning, so she opened the window of our second floor classroom.

This was a fine idea and the incoming breeze felt good, but it so happened that the second graders were outside on recess during that time and the playground was located on our side of the building. Some of the kids were playing against the red brick wall, directly below the window.

The rambunctious kids were a little too noisy, and finally Mrs. Akin stuck her head out the window and yelled, "Shut up down there!"

That worked for five minutes, but then the volume increased so that it was even louder than before.

"I said to shut up," she yelled again out the window. She had lost her patience and was frustrated.

The preoccupied second graders ignored the elderly lady scolding them, and they continued with their noisy play.

In a huff, Mrs. Akin muttered, "Be right back," and she stormed out of the room. I figured she was fed up and needed her cigar.

A few minutes later, though, she walked back into the room carrying a five gallon bucket that was halfway filled with water.

It was obviously heavy, but that wasn't going to deter her from achieving her goal.

The kids were still noisy down below.

Mrs. Akin looked out the window and then turned and gave us a wink and a smile. She lifted the bucket and dumped the water out the window and onto the children below.

Their playground laughter turned into shrieks.

"I warned them," she said triumphantly.

She picked up where she left off with Thurber. Not a peep was heard from the playground outside for the rest of the class period.

Where Am I

There are few things in life that I want more than to be healed. I am hoping for a cure. I hope that I can live long enough to see and play with my grandkids. I hope I can have a comfortable retirement. There is no certainty with Parkinson's, though.

While waiting for a cure, I'm watching my body slow down; perhaps even scarier, I'm watching my brain slow down. What is it like to see my "old age" approaching with rapid acceleration?

When I'm off, my gait is a shuffle. My long legs (I am nearly 6 feet 3 inches tall) want to take big steps, but my brain has trouble making the legs move. I can force my legs to take big steps, but I really have to stop and think "big step, big step, big step" one step at a time. If there is clutter on the floor, or when walking through a narrow passage or doorway, it is even more difficult.

Balance is a big issue for me as well. Standing on one leg to put on a pair of pants or a shoe is nearly impossible. If I close both eyes and lose whatever reference point I'm using to retain a sense of being upright, I easily tip over. My wife prefers to keep the bedroom totally dark at night, and it makes it very difficult to walk across the floor to the bathroom.

I have only fallen four times as of this writing—twice at work and twice at home—but I have caught myself from falling (generally by grabbing furniture on the way down) numerous times.

Speech continues to be very difficult for me. I'm at my best when I'm reading something aloud, though in the past few months even that has become more challenging. I'll open my mouth to speak and words won't come out. This morning, for example, when the furnace repairman came to our house to fix a problem, I wanted to explain that the air conditioning was working fine but the heater wasn't. I began a sentence with "The" ... and it literally took 20 seconds for the next word ("AC") to come out.

I have seen video footage of myself speaking, and it is embarrassing. My lips go into contortions, my eyes blink frequently, and my face reminds me of someone who is in the middle of being swallowed by a giant octopus. It's not pretty.

I bit my lip eating breakfast this morning. It seems that I do that frequently. There's something wrong with the timing of how my mouth, cheeks, and tongue move the food from my lips back to my esophagus. At least, it seems as though things get out of rhythm, out of sync, and my teeth clamp down at the wrong time.

I am dyskinetic as I'm writing this. My head can't stay still; my neck and mouth are twitching; my shoulders are rolling and rocking; and it's amazing that I can even type anything. I tend to be more dyskinetic when I am "on"—i.e., at my best—and not dyskinetic when I am "off."

Cognitively, things aren't going so well. Oh, the creative side of my brain still functions. The executive functioning part of the brain— problem solving, organizing, and trying to make connections with gobs of data—gets confused. Decision making is tough for me now.

I used to be a software engineer, writing complex computer software. If you know software, I wrote code for compilers and operating systems. Yeah, that was real stuff. I did this type of work for over twenty years. Year after year, I would be given awards, bonuses, stock options, and promotions.

Then, the past several years, my performance rapidly declined, decaying like a tooth in a bottle of Coca Cola. Until that point in time, I had loved going into work. I would wake up every morning, excited about the upcoming day in the office. I was eager to tackle the next big problem. That was my thing.

Then, suddenly, almost overnight, the work became difficult. I was dropping details. My quality suffered. My quantity suffered. Because I wasn't doing well, work stopped being fun. I tried increasing my hours so that I could get more done, but that didn't help.

My employer tried putting me on long-term disability for cognitive impairment, but the employer's disability insurance company had me tested by an "independent" psychologist who ruled that I was fine, not cognitively impaired. Interestingly, though he put me through six or seven hours of testing, the simplistic tests did not really reflect the type of work with which I was having difficulty.

The insurance company denied my disability claim. Because my performance at work was not acceptable, my employer had no choice but to terminate my employment. With no income and no primary disability insurance, life became interesting. We hired an attorney and appealed the decision, and—just days ago, a year after we had been denied—the insurance company changed its mind.

Yes, it has been a financial struggle. But you know what? God tells us to rejoice always. Jesus himself tells us to be cheerful, regardless of what the world is doing to us or what we are experiencing.

> In the world you will have trouble.
> But take heart! I have overcome the world.
>
> —John 16:33b

The hope that we have in Christ is not a thing of chance; it's not something that we need to worry about happening or not. It's a given. In Ephesians, Paul writes that the hope of salvation is our helmet. The world can beat us up all it wants to, but our helmet—the hope of salvation—protects us. The reason we can have hope—the reason we can have certainty—is because of Christ's salvation. Jesus Christ already fought and won the battle for us. If Jesus is our Lord, the blood he shed on the cross has atoned for our sins and his resurrection has given us eternal life.

The hope that we have in Christ is not a wish. It's a guarantee. The hope that I have in Christ is what gives me the ability to get out of bed in the morning, knowing it's going to be a great day. This Parkinson's thing is only temporary, for however long I have on earth. I can laugh at it because, in the big picture, my hope does not rest on the things of this world. My hope rests in Christ.

Telling Stories

The more I write down stories of things that happened in my life as a child and as an adult, the more I understand how my life ties to my kids' lives. The stories form a tapestry of life and history and provide glimpses into my heart that capture the essence of what I believe to be important in life.

The more I write, the more I remember, and the more I remember, the more I appreciate the sense of family that my parents have given me. My parents told me tales of their parents, and some of the tales they told had been passed down from their grandparents. My kids have heard some of these tales as well, and their understanding of family heritage is blossoming.

For my children, the stories are comforting; as they hear about some of the silly situations and tough times in which I found myself, they can see that there is hope even in times when they encounter adversity.

During a recent Christmas week, as my family was vacationing on North Carolina's Outer Banks, my youngest daughter Laura came down with a nasty stomach illness. She asked me if I would tell her some stories, and I was delighted to have the opportunity. As a parent, I find great cheer in hearing one of my children say, "Please tell me a story from when you were a kid."

I told her a few stories, some that I have already written down and some that have yet to see ink. Though our story time together didn't cure her, it brought a smile to a face that I hadn't seen smile for the previous two days.

After telling the stories, I asked her if she would like me to read to her. She nodded. I ran upstairs, where everyone else was playing a board game, and I asked, "Hey, I need something to read to Laura. Any ideas?"

My oldest daughter Alex spoke up immediately. "How about reading something from the Bible?" Now how cool is that, when a teenager suggests reading the Bible!

The Bible that I had brought with me on the trip was *The Message*, and I grabbed it off my night stand and went back down to Laura's room. Her eyes sparkled when she saw that I was going to read from the Bible.

I stroked her hair as I read to her, trying anything to make her comfortable. My heart ached for her.

I started with Psalm 63, and I was reading it aloud with feeling and compassion until I got to the line that Eugene Peterson translated as "prime rib and gravy" (the NIV says "richest of foods"), and as I read it I could see Laura's face turning green. I should have skipped that verse.

There is something transforming in a relationship when two people—even father and daughter—spend time together. As I read and told stories to Laura, I thought back to when my parents would read to me when I was sick. I know that someday Laura will have the opportunity to tell family stories or read to others who just need someone to be there; and I know that she will be blessed in the same ways that I was blessed in our time together.

You know what? I don't have to wait for one of my kids to be sick to be able to do this again. The opportunity is there almost every evening! What a privilege to be able to spend time together like this.

See, telling stories is only partly about helping connect to the past and to see our lives in the context of our heritage; telling stories is also about establishing and strengthening relationships.

The next time you're about to turn on the television, try this instead: "Hey kids, instead of watching television tonight, let me tell you a story about something that happened to me when I was your age."

Everybody's got a story to tell, but not everyone enjoys telling stories. Maybe you want to flip through an old family photo album or scrapbook. Tell your child his birth story. Share a story of something funny or embarrassing that happened to you as a child. Spend time together. You'll be glad you did.

In the Trenches

January has always been a tough month for me, and this month is no different than the four dozen previous Januaries I have waded. Four dozen! That number almost boggles my mind. At least it's not twelve dozen ... that would be, uh, positively gross.

January is when we descend the mountain from Christmas and we stay in the valley—or the trenches—until Easter approaches. I love Christmas and I love Easter, and sometimes the gap between the two is a little tough to handle.

Yet, I also embrace this time. This is real life. This is where it matters. This is where the rubber meets the road. This is where faith gets a chance to exercise, the opportunity to stretch its arms and legs and play some hardball in the game of life.

The air is cold; the skies are gray; the days are short; and we are called to rejoice. "Rejoice always, even in January," Paul might have written.

The chickens this time of year, when we let them out of their coop to run around the yard, scurry over to places where fallen leaves have accumulated. They methodically and thoroughly turn over the leaves, looking for bugs or worms to eat. The fact that it's January doesn't prevent them from looking for good stuff.

My heart needs to be doing the same thing. I need to be looking for the good things.

It's January: I just spent three days with two nephews and a niece, playing games and laughing more than I've laughed in months. I have a niece who is convinced that I named a character in one of my recent manuscripts after her; I have a nephew who loves to play Pigmania with Uncle Joel; and I have another nephew who exclaimed (during an intense Capture the Flag game), "Wow, you're fast, Uncle Joel!"

Our church orchestra played with the choir for the anthem at church yesterday; what a joy it is to play in the orchestra! We rehearse on Sunday evenings and I always look forward to it.

I talked with countless friends at church as well ... each one a blessing to me.

Sure, there are some difficult, sticky issues going on in my life at the moment. Should I dwell on them? No. Yes, they'll get addressed. The things to set my mind on, though, are the joyful moments that God places before me every day.

When I stop fretting and start looking around, there are a ton of blessings each day.

It's my choice. I can look in the mirror, whine and pout, and feel sorry for myself; or I can look up to heaven, see God, and say, "Thank you."

I choose the latter. Come to think of it, I love Januaries. Don't you?

I have to admit that it's not all rosy having Parkinson's Disease; it's not all fun and games. There are times (like right now) where I get depressed. Oh, I don't get depressed too often, but it happens.

It happens to you, too, doesn't it? If it's any consolation, even people who aren't battling illness can get depressed. Sometimes the depression is a short-lived, temporary mindset; sometimes, though, it can be serious and debilitating. Depression can be caused from medications; depression can be caused by external circumstances (stress, relationship issues, etc.); and depression can be caused by chemical imbalances in the body.

If you are frequently depressed, I encourage you to seek help. Talk to your doctor or pastor and you will be pointed in the right direction.

Why do I get depressed? In my heart I know God is here with me; in my heart I know he loves me, is taking care of me, and won't forget about me. I know that spiritually.

The crazy thing is that I also know, both physically and rationally, that God is holding me in his arms. There really is a God.

"How can that be?" you ask. "How can you feel physically held by God?"

I don't know. I just do. The same comfort, the same relief, and the same joy that comes from an enormous hug from someone whom you love very much—those same things are present, 24x7 every day of the year.

Yet, even with that certainty, God allows me to feel depressed. Maybe it's just a gentle reminder that I need to depend on him for everything; I need to lean on him.

At any rate, I don't stay depressed for long.

Do I believe happiness is a choice? Yes, I do. That doesn't mean that depression can't settle in like a fog in a harbor. Where is the lighthouse that will prevent you from crashing into the rocky shore? It's in Psalm 63. It's in Habakkuk 3. It's in John 3:16. It's throughout God's Word, where verse after verse portrays God's love for us.

Remember, the Creator of the Universe also made you. He who became flesh and dwelt among us also died on the cross for you. He knows your name. He loves you and he wants to help you.

> Come to me, all you who are weary and burdened,
> and I will give you rest. Take my yoke upon you
> and learn from me, for I am gentle and humble in
> heart, and you will find rest for your souls.
> For my yoke is easy and my burden is light.
>
> —Matthew 11:28–30

> He heals the brokenhearted and binds up their wounds.
>
> —Psalm 147:3

> Cast all your anxiety on him because he cares for you.
>
> —1 Peter 5:7

For I am convinced that neither death nor life, neither angels nor demons, neither the present nor the future, nor any powers, neither height nor depth, nor anything else in all creation, will be able to separate us from the love of God that is in Christ Jesus our Lord.

—Romans 8:38–39

Who Are You?

Do you identify yourself by your job? Are you a lawyer, a doctor, or a college entrance exam proctor? Are you a pharmacist, a radiologist, or a farmer-turned-anthropologist? Maybe you work in a daycare or at the state fair, or perhaps your job is to do people's hair. Are you a rock star? Do you lay tar? Do you play honky tonk in a college town bar? You might be a stay-at-home mom or stay-at-home dad. Perhaps you play tuba to cheer people up when they're sad. Or you might work in a watch factory where you sit around all day making faces.

So, when people ask you who you are, do you identify yourself by your job?

"Hi, I'm Joel. I'm a writer, but ... but ... I did develop software for almost twenty-five years. Really, honest, I used to have a real job."

Maybe you prefer to answer that question with your favorite hobby. I'm a tuba player; I'm a football coach. How about you? Maybe you play the violin or prune azaleas or send text messages until your thumbs are about ready to fall off. "Hi, I'm Dexter the texter." Maybe you're an amateur singer, or perhaps you are a hobbyist who enjoys spending free time as a seamstress or tailor (someone who sews, versus a sewer). Are you a blogger, a clogger, or a mountainside logger?

What's your hobby? Is that how you identify yourself?

"Hi, I'm Joel. I caught a seven pound largemouth bass once. I kept it and it's in the trunk of my car. Wanna see it?"

We also like to identify ourselves by our collegiate affiliations, and we tend to imply that our school's successes are a direct link back to us.

"Hi, I'm Joel. I went to Nebraska. We've won the football national championship five times. How about you?" That tends to be a really popular way to introduce yourself.

An alternative is to identify yourself by your family.

"I'm a dad of four."

"Oh really? Well I'm a dad of five."

"Five? That's nothing. I'm a dad of seventeen."

Seventeen sounds like a lot of kids until you consider that one of the world's most famous composers fathered 20 children. As amazing as that was (and is), the number of kids he had is not usually the first thing people think of when they hear the name Johann Sebastian Bach.

We even identify ourselves by our kids' accomplishments sometime.

"Hi, I'm Joel. I have four kids, and my oldest daughter won a goldfish at our church's fall festival when she was three."

Do you identify yourself with an illness? "Hi, I'm Joel. I have Parkinson's." By the way, that's a great way to introduce yourself to people at a party. It sets the tone, gets everybody in a sort of happy mindset, and makes for a great evening ... not.

The problem with all of this is that we are trying to identify ourselves by our accomplishments, someone else's accomplishments, or with sympathy-seeking labels. We are proud of what we do, where we've been, or what we have, and sometimes (or often) we cross the boundaries of being self-absorbed, self-possessed, and self-obsessed.

What if, instead, we identified ourselves with something eternal, something that will last forever?

"Who are you?"

"I am a child of God."

It's not bragging. It's not lifting up yourself. It's merely saying that God's love for you is more important to you than all the things you do.

You are loved because you are a child of God.

You have value because you are a child of God.

Your worth has nothing to do with what you've done, where you've been, whom you know, or what you have. Your worth has everything to do with the fact that God created you and he loves you.

Whether it's how you identify yourself to others or not, don't ever forget it. You are a beloved child of God.

Perseverance

Most of you will agree that almost everything in life worth pursuing demands effort. You can't build a relationship that is one-sided and focused on yourself. You have to work to get to know the other person. You can't (generally) get a good job without putting in the effort to study and work hard at school. You can't master a musical instrument without making it a priority, which often means giving up other things you would like to do as well.

Sometimes, I think, the thing that is worth pursuing is life itself. So you're young, you have this incurable disease, and as far as you can tell your life is going to continue. You can choose to be miserable, or you can choose to accept it and make the best of each day.

The hard things to deal with include facing the fact that your future has changed. Maybe you won't live in a comfortable retirement; maybe you won't be traveling or taking on new hobbies or whatever it was that you were planning to do; and maybe you won't be living the long life that you've been planning since you were a child.

The worst thing you can do is to sit on the couch and mope. If you can do anything positive at all, do it.

Maybe you've lost your job and there's no hope of getting another. How can you spend your time? Well, for one, you could go to a rest home for seniors and spend time talking with, feeding, or entertaining the people there. Maybe you can work with underprivileged youth who have never had a chance to make it in life. You can make a difference, somewhere, somehow.

The thing is that you've got to push yourself. With Parkinson's Disease, it's so hard to find the energy; it's hard to be "on" all the time (or at least at the right times). You've got to do what you can do. Do a little; then try a little more; and then try yet even more.

Don't give up the race, ever. Don't ever quit. Don't ever say, "I'm finished."

Let God decide when he's done with you. Let God decide when it's time to call you home.

Here's good news for you. When your days on earth are done, that's not the end. That's the beginning.

> The Lord is my shepherd,
> I shall not be in want.
> He makes me lie down in green pastures,
> he leads me beside quiet waters,
> he restores my soul.
>
> He guides me in paths of
> righteousness for his name's sake.
> Even though I walk through the valley
> of the shadow of death,
> I will fear no evil,
> for you are with me;
> your rod and your staff,
> they comfort me.
>
> You prepare a table before me
> in the presence of my enemies.
> You anoint my head with oil;
> my cup overflows.
>
> Surely goodness and love will follow me
> all the days of my life,
> and I will dwell in the house of the Lord
> forever.
>
> —Psalm 23

When It's Dark

We can't possibly grasp what was going through the mind of Jesus as he slowly inched toward a painful, humiliating death on the cross.

Jesus—fully God but also fully man, who on the cross was still capable of experiencing every emotion known by humankind—had been abandoned by his close friends. Peter, the one whom Jesus had nicknamed "The Rock," had explicitly denied Jesus three times. John stayed around, lurking in the shadows and trying hard to remain unnoticed.

The disciples were scared and confused. This small band of men had been prepared, they thought, to follow their Messiah on his ascension as leader and king as he conquered the Romans and restored Israel.

They were weary of the "old life" and were excited about this new kingdom that Jesus had described.

On that first Good Friday, the disciples reached a chasm, a canyon, that seemed impassable. This gap separated their old (and current) life from their new life. Their leader was crucified; their hope was shattered. There seemed to be no way across.

They didn't understand that it was the cross itself that was the bridge across the chasm. They wouldn't really understand this until Pentecost, when the Holy Spirit came and filled them.

Have you faced any chasms in your life? What chasm are you staring down today?

The chasm is great, but there's good news. A bridge has been built that will allow you to walk across. The bridge is the cross.

You still have to walk. It's your choice.

On this side of Pentecost, we don't really know what the disciples went through. The Holy Spirit gives us hope and courage. The disciples didn't have that on the day Jesus was crucified.

We have a source of hope, a source of peace, a source of joy and goodness and strength and courage.

When all is dark, when that chasm seems too great, when it seems that there is no way out—we still have hope.

It's dark. It's dreary out there. But Sunday's coming.

Where, O Death, Is Now Thy Sting?

*O*f all the lyrics traditionally sung around Easter, the line that always hits home for me is "Where, O Death, is now thy sting?" from Charles Wesley's song "Christ the Lord Is Risen Today."

Yesterday was April 24, 2011. Easter Sunday! For years, this has been my favorite day. It's not just the music; it's not just the uplifting messages at church; but it's also the hope, the promise, that this brief life on earth isn't all there is.

I've had a bad cough, coupled with a head cold, for the past three or four days, and that has led to fitful sleep at night.

Saturday night—the night before Easter—while sleeping, I managed to wrench something in my back. I don't know what it was or how it happened, but I awoke unable to turn over.

It was a struggle trying to get out of bed Sunday morning. I sort of inched my way to the edge of the bed. I'm not quite sure how I did it, but by the time I finally got out of bed, I was already worn out and the day hadn't even started yet!

It also took a long time for my meds to kick in, which meant that my shower was in "slow motion" ...

You ought to see me try to button a shirt when I'm still "off" in the morning. You know how, when you play backyard football, the defense will count "3 Mississippi's" before rushing the quarterback? Yesterday morning I needed about 5 Mississippi's per button.

So it was stressful getting ready for church. On my way out the door, I remembered ... my tuba! I reached to pick it up. Ouch! I had forgotten about my back.

By the time I was in the car and on my way to church, my body felt battered. It was as though I had lost a fight to Dirty Harry. "Do you feel lucky? Well do ya, punk?"

But you know what? It was Easter Sunday.

My body had been beaten, but my heart said, "Let's go!"

It didn't matter that I had a cough or cold; it didn't matter that I struggled to pick up my tuba for each piece we played; and it didn't matter that I was tired and fighting the temptation to sleep.

What mattered? My heart is what mattered—or more specifically, the joy through Christ that is in my heart.

The joy I felt in church on Sunday wasn't something I dreamed up. The joy that I felt was a gift. Namely, the joy came from Christ's resurrection.

Life is hard—whether it's a cough, physical discomfort, lack of sleep, Parkinson's Disease or choose your favorite illness—but the resurrection says that there is more than just the mortal life we live here.

Influential German theologian Dietrich Bonhoeffer was held prisoner in a German concentration camp near the end of World War II. In April of 1945, as he was conducting a worship service in the camp, German soldiers came and ordered him to "make ready" and to come with them, the standard pronouncement for one who was about to be executed.

The next day, Bonhoeffer was led to the gallows. Various accounts from witnesses all agree that Bonhoeffer was at peace and that his face expressed joy. In his last recorded words, he stated that this was the end—but for him, the beginning—of life. He was executed less than a week before Allied forces reached and freed the camp.

Why was Bonhoeffer joyful? He grasped the hope of Easter.

On Good Friday, Satan said, "You have no way out. I win."

On Easter Sunday, God shouted, "You're wrong, Satan," and he made a move that Satan didn't see coming. "Checkmate!"

It doesn't matter that I showed up at church feeling as though I had been hit by a freight train. It was a joyful day! I went home after church and spent much of the afternoon in bed. This morning, I'm still coughing.

Do I feel great? No. Am I happy? Yes. Am I joyful? Absolutely!

Also by Joel Schnoor

I Laid an Egg on Aunt Ruth's Head

Conquering English and ~~It's~~ Its Ruthless Ways

I Laid an Egg on Aunt Ruth's Head: Conquering English and Its Ruthless Ways might be the perfect grammar supplement for teens who already have the basics but could use a little polish. Most adults should also find it useful. Author Joel Schnoor entertains while he instructs through humorous stories of his Great Aunt Ruth.
— Cathy Duffy Reviews

Clever, witty, and surprisingly edifying, *I Laid an Egg on Aunt Ruth's Head* is a can't miss literary treat for true lovers of the English language ... Schnoor's insightful, amusing approach successfully breathes new life into what is typically viewed as a rather mundane subject.
— Apex Reviews

I am not a fan of cute grammar books that seem designed to put down those who make common mistakes. Schnoor's book is definitely not that. He is a kind, considerate, funny teacher who wants only for his students to improve, not to feel bad because of all they don't know.
— Pam Nelson, Raleigh News and Observer

This is a funny book but it covers some serious grammar.
— M.S. Hahn, Teacher

Available from www.GennesaretPress.com

CPSIA information can be obtained
at www.ICGtesting.com
Printed in the USA
FFOW04n1843150216
21413FF

9 780984 554126